W9-BMP-043

GET...
SUDDENLY SLIM!®

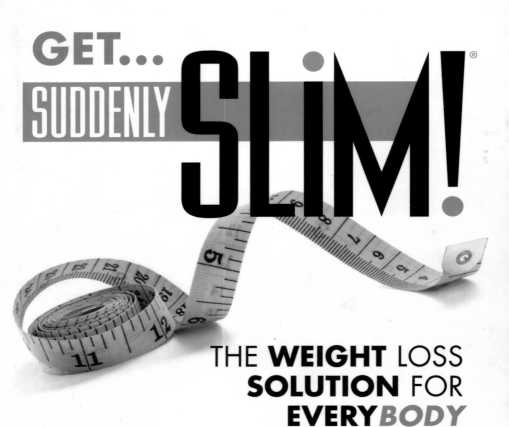

THE **WEIGHT** LOSS **SOLUTION** FOR **EVERY**BODY

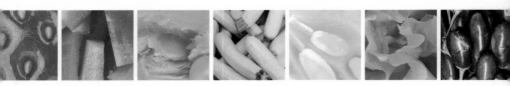

LEE CAUSEY

WEIGHT LOSS PIONEER & CREATOR OF THE WORLD'S FIRST DIET SHAKE

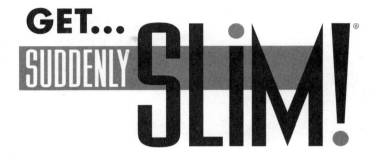

GET...
SUDDENLY SLIM!®

THE **WEIGHT** LOSS **SOLUTION** FOR **EVERY**BODY

LEE CAUSEY

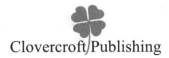

Clovercroft Publishing

Get Suddenly Slim

©2016 by Lee Causey

Published by Clovercroft Publishing, Franklin, Tennessee.

Published in association with Larry Carpenter of Christian Book Services, LLC. www.christianbookservices.com

Contributing Writing by Sarah Karger

Cover and Interior Design by Lori Newman

Editing by Adept Content Solutions

Printed in the United States of America

978-1-942557-47-0

DEDICATION

To Anita Causey, my beautiful and loyal wife of over 55 years, without your support and belief in me this would never have been possible.

To Nigel Branson, President and Co-Founder of FirstFitness Nutrition, whose business leadership, work ethic, and commitment to building a great company that has made a positive difference in thousands of people's lives.

To #TeamFFN distributors, medical professionals, and FFN employees who have been so dedicated to the mission and vision of FirstFitness Nutrition, bringing health, wellness, and a better way of life to the world.

TABLE OF CONTENTS

FOREWORD

It has always been my personal and medical opinion that if a person wants to have exceptional and vibrant health in order to be disease free, a person must invest and commit many years into the studies, applications, and principles associated with nutrition. Sound nutrition, supplementation, and exercise are necessary and critical in order to achieve a sustained state of wellness that results in true physical, mental, emotional, and spiritual longevity. It is imperative that we understand that all living and healing processes are bound to one another through the workings of nutrients.

It has been shown repeatedly that the foods individuals consume are strong indicators and most accurate predictors of both quality and length of life, reproductive health, mental clarity, and most importantly disease anomalies. For the past fifty years, the American diet has confirmed through demonstration and substantiation that the quality of our present-day nutrition is less valuable than that of our ancestors. Because of our poor quality of nutrition, the American people are holding themselves hostage living with lower standards of health.

Having practiced and taught in the public health sector of infectious diseases, I was, like many medical professionals, relying on prescription drugs as the primary tool for health issues. I was amazed to find volumes of published medical research showing botanicals, nutrients, and phytonutrients were used in the place of certain medicines to help correct various metabolic imbalances, which resulted in the reversal of acute and chronic degenerative diseases. In 1930, a Norwegian homeopath, Dr.

Victor G. Rocine stated, *"If we eat wrongly, no doctor can cure us; if we eat rightly, no doctor is needed."* Nutrition has been used in medicine since 460 B.C. when Hippocrates, the "father of medicine," stated that *"Food is your best medicine, and the best foods are the best medicines."* How fortunate for us today that nearly 50 years ago a humble humanitarian by the name of Lee Causey developed a passion and concern for promoting human welfare through exercise, supplements, and correct nutrition.

My first encounter with FirstFitness Nutrition was through an acquaintance from church who had lost 90 pounds in 6 months on the *Suddenly Slim* Weight Loss Program. I lost 18 pounds in 10 days and went on to lose 57 pounds in 7 weeks and have kept the weight off. During the 14 years that I have known Lee Causey, I have served on his medical and scientific advisory board and worked alongside him assisting with several product development projects. Because of his many years of expertise in nutrition and supplementation, Lee Causey has helped thousands of people to reverse chronic health issues, resulting in a better quality of life. In the theater of health and wellness, Lee is considered one of the most knowledgeable pioneers in the health and wellness industry.

The information in the *Get Suddenly Slim* book is insightful, interesting, fascinating, and most importantly, helpful. The reader will find that a person does not have to be overweight or obese to be nutrient deficient. If you are personally or know someone experiencing health related issues mostly due to being overweight or obese, I would highly suggest reading this book by Lee Causey on nutrition as the first approach to improving your health. I agree with Lee's direct approach as to why *"the struggle is real"* when it comes to poor nutrition as one of the chief causes of creating a compromised immune system resulting in debilitating diseases such as cardiovascular, diabetes, arthritis, and cancer.

I'm very humble to have been asked to write this Foreword, and I know reading *Get Suddenly Slim* by Lee Causey will educate and, most importantly, create a mindset for whole-body transformation.

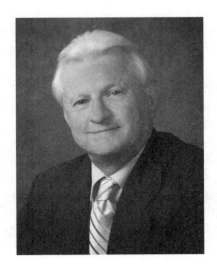

BYRON R. COON, DrPH, PhD

PREFACE

My partnership with weight loss pioneer and health and wellness expert Lee Causey began in 1989, when he founded his new company FirstFitness Nutrition. He invited me on a crusade to change the world with his revolutionary inner body and colon cleanser Reneú®. After the successful introduction of that product, Lee started producing a new line of weight loss products. For the first 10 years of my career with Lee Causey and FirstFitness Nutrition, I lived an exciting life. A health and fitness enthusiast in my own right, we had a thriving company, and I was traveling around the country introducing people to the products and our business opportunity. Life was good.

However, one morning it all changed for me. I was in a terrible motorcycle accident. I severed the ACL and PCL ligaments in my left knee, along with my ACL, PCL, and MCL ligaments in my right knee. Confined to a wheelchair for almost five months, the surplus of medications I was prescribed, including cortisone, steroids, and pain meds, left me with an appetite nothing short of ravenous. I just couldn't stop eating. No longer having the ability to work off even some of the enormous surplus of calories I was consuming, I gained 94 pounds in just under a year.

"I JUST COULDN'T STOP EATING!"

We go through our life, never expecting the day to come when our world is flipped upside down. There I was living the high life one morning, and by the afternoon, I was physically handicapped. Forget exercise—I couldn't even walk for five months! I was unable to do almost anything without the assistance of someone else.

After time my body healed, but I was left with 94 pounds, as a daily reminder of all I had endured. For the first time in my life, I truly understood the sheer pain and suffering overweight people felt.

I was angry. My stress levels were at an all-time high. I replaced all of my clothes with baggy and oversized options to hide my body. I turned down invitations to social events. To add insult to injury, there I was the president of a weight loss and wellness company, giving presentations and promoting our products as an obese person. I could hear people under their breath snickering, wondering if I even used the products myself. It was at that moment I thought I would never bounce back.

You're probably wondering why I didn't get on Lee Causey's weight loss products. I did. In fact, that's what I told Lee. But really, I would start on a Monday morning and would quit by lunchtime. In our meetings, I remember he would ask me if I was following the weight loss program and sticking to menu, both of us knowing full well I wasn't. You see, it doesn't matter who helps you if you aren't willing to help yourself. Until I was ready to personally improve my body and health, I would continue to waste what little effort I put forth by filling my body with overprocessed and toxic foods every other meal.

One day, I went to the doctor for a physical and was forced to face the harsh reality of my circumstance. He declared with certainty that if I didn't lose 40 to 50 pounds, and quickly, it would be detrimental to my life. I would follow in my father's and grandfather's footsteps. My father had a life-long struggle with his heart and eventually passed away a few years ago from congestive heart failure and blood cancer. My grandfather died at 42 from a heart attack. This was my wake-up call. At this stage in my life, I had 4 kids, and I couldn't bear to leave them fatherless. I knew I had to act now. It was then that my "Why" hit me square in the face.

I had to stop feeling sorry for myself, stop playing the victim, and actually commit to losing this weight. I started on *Suddenly Slim* and in the first 6 months, I lost 40 pounds and went on to lose a total of 94 pounds. Sticking to the *Suddenly Slim* Program, I am proud to tell you, I've maintained this weight loss for more than 10 years. I have continued to be a product of the products, and I'm a firm believer that the *Suddenly Slim* Weight Loss Program will be your weight loss solution, too. Thank you, Lee Causey, for personally helping me achieve freedom from the despair of obesity.

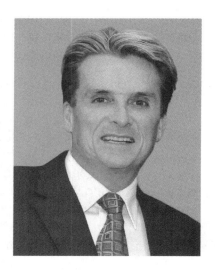

NIGEL BRANSON
FirstFitness Nutrition
President & Co-Founder

INTRODUCTION

As humans, we have done incredible, spectacular things on this earth, things our ancestors and their ancestors before them never dreamed were possible. Largely due to the human spirit and its growth, we as a people are continually building on top of these accomplishments. But for the first time, I see our potential as a human race being thwarted. Despite our abundant spirit, we are placing shackles on our overwhelming potential thanks to the restrictions today's food has placed on our bodies.

I've written this book to help the hundreds of millions of people who face these shackles every day. This book is for those who wake up looking for a weight-loss solution that actually works; people who are sick and tired of being sick and tired. This book is for those people who are desperately looking for a solution to their problems, and willing to take action to put a stop to this epidemic, by making themselves and their family's health a priority.

We weren't placed on this earth to be anemic, feeble, and helpless beings just making do with what we've been given. Our role on this earth is to excel at every opportunity and leave this world a better place than when we came into it.

Many people have either seen or heard of the movie, *Super-Size Me*, about one man's social experiment, incorporating McDonald's into his diet 3 times a day for 30 days. His cholesterol skyrocketed, he developed an addiction, and his weight, and proportionately, his body fat shot up in just 30 days. This is to say nothing of the people who have been eating this way for years. Fast-food chains like McDonald's have infiltrated our lives and trained us to rely on their fast food.

However, and I want to be very clear on this subject—I do not blame you. My justified criticism rests at the feet of the food industry, which I've named Food Inc. This is aptly named for its shortcomings on serving its customers. It is a business, first and foremost, with the sole purpose of making as much money as possible with a growing concern for its bottom line. As long as it continues to grow, it cares not what repercussions arise for you, even if your waistline grows in tandem with that bottom line. It employs deceitful and malicious tactics in building its empire to ensure success, which ensures you, the consumer, will be faced with a multitude of problems, both physically and financially.

This body is the only one we get; we have to take care of it, and this book will teach you how.

Having been in the health and wellness industry for more than 50 years, my career started back in my competitive bodybuilding days. Working alongside personal and professional friend, Arnold Schwarzenegger, I cultivated a burning desire to make a lasting, positive difference in those around me through health and wellness. This is my life's calling. I will do everything in my power to navigate you to the same success I've helped millions of other people achieve. Through changing your lifestyle and your body, you will achieve a healthier, slimmer, and happier life.

"THIS BODY IS THE ONLY ONE WE GET; WE HAVE TO TAKE CARE OF IT, AND THIS BOOK WILL TEACH YOU HOW."

My inspiration for this path all started in a small town in north Florida in the 1940s. My youngest brother, Robert, had contracted polio and fell extremely ill. As the disease attacked his legs, he wasn't expected to live. To this day, I can still hear his suffering-filled screams as my mother was left with little to do to relieve his excruciating pain than attempt massage therapy.

Thank God, Robert lived, but he was paralyzed from the waist down. As the eldest son I quite literally had to bear the weight of this debilitating disease on my shoulders. It became my responsibility to carry Robert everywhere we went.

As polio was very contagious, I too contracted the disease, but by some miracle was left with only a minor weakness in my back. This firsthand suffering, not only of my brother, but of my mother as she sat helplessly watching her child writhe in agony, inspired my path in life to devote myself to helping others not only become, but to stay healthy. I desired to make a lasting impression on the health industry.

After receiving a full football scholarship to the University of Florida, my initial inclination was to go into medicine. After all, they help people who are sick. But I quickly learned that doctors today didn't educate patients on proactive health practices but were entirely reactive. I couldn't thrive in a world where I was forced to wait and treat people once they became sick, like my brother, or worse. No, I had to educate people before they let ailments control their existence.

At the time, I believed the answer to health was exercise. So naturally I threw myself entirely into that field. I became a nationally competitive bodybuilder, and Anita, my wife, was a beauty contestant. Our life centered on health, wellness, and fitness through exercise and nutrition. I developed exercise equipment along with nutritional programs to encourage people to improve their lives, just as I had. As a result, I was one of the first people in the United States to open a chain of modern-day health clubs. Starting with practically nothing, I was a millionaire by the age of 25. But more important than my wealth, I was blessed with the opportunity to positively affect people's lives through health.

My first major marketing discovery in the health and fitness industry was the realization that people were not really that interested in their overall health; they just wanted to lose weight. Being healthy was just a side effect of shedding fat. This led me to develop the world's first diet shake. Testing it on one of my gym members resulted in an incredible weight loss of 29 pounds in 30 days. The success of that product was phenomenal, and diet shakes continue to be the number-one selling health and wellness product to date.

Much later in my life, I contracted a rare virus that drove me to over use antibiotics, which caused me to gain over 100 pounds in only 4 months. While modern medicine is something we cannot renounce for very obvious reasons, I now know I was filling my body with toxic chemicals. It wasn't until I discovered a small paperback called *Rational Fasting* by Arnold Ehret that discussed the benefits of cleansing and detoxification that my life changed, again. Through the use of many different botanical extracts and herbs highly regarded by the book, I lost all of the weight I had gained in just 5 months.

At last, I had discovered the real secret of losing weight and keep it off: cleansing and detoxification! I wanted to share this with the world. Along with the expert assistance from trusted friend and nutritional scientist, Dr. Richard Kaufman, I created the first cleansing and detoxification product, an all-in-one capsule called Reneú®.

Over the past 26 years Reneú® has proved to be paramount to overall health, and an essential piece of the foundation to a successful weight loss program. Cleansing and detoxification, as I discuss in further detail in the book, supercharge your weight loss allowing your body to absorb nutrients it lacked for so long, and flush toxins, as well as, fat out of the body. Paired with the other products in my *Suddenly Slim* Weight Loss Programs, you will finally lose the weight. The vast nutritional knowledge I've accumulated over the years through my ongoing research will help you keep it off, something that other weight loss programs can't claim.

I am thrilled you've decided to take the first step. Knowledge is a powerful tool, and it will sustain you well beyond the weight loss of our *Suddenly Slim* Weight Loss Programs.

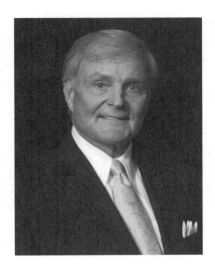

LEE CAUSEY
Weight Loss Pioneer &
Creator of the World's First Diet Shake

CHAPTER 1

WHY WE **GET FAT**

Have you ever gotten out of bed and looked in the mirror one day to find you look ... different? It's as if you gained weight overnight. Your face has gotten plump, rounder. Your favorite jeans no longer fit like they used to. They are starting to push your flab over the top creating that dreaded muffin top. Well, if this is you, welcome to the club. At last count, the Center for Disease Control classified 69% of Americans overweight. **Sixty-nine percent**. Of the more than 2/3 of our population facing the same epidemic that is staring back at you in the mirror, just over half, 35%, are obese. To be classified as obese, an individual must weigh more than 20% of what is considered to be normal.

What's normal, you ask? Good question. While every*body* is different, traditionally a normal level of body fat is identified using your Body Mass Index/BMI. Simply put, this cross references your height and weight to reach a percentage of body fat. Any percentage over 24.9 is considered to be overweight. Calculating your BMI can be a great way to assess your individual situation, but it's not without issue. Some people are genetically heavier, some carry more muscle than others, but as a general rule of thumb, it's definitely where we should start.

BMI | BODY MASS INDEX CHART

Height	Weight		
	Normal	**Overweight**	**Obese**
4' 10"	91 to 118 lbs.	119 to 142 lbs.	143 to 186 lbs.
4' 11"	94 to 123 lbs.	124 to 147 lbs.	148 to 193 lbs.
5' 0"	97 to 127 lbs.	128 to 152 lbs.	153 to 199 lbs.
5' 1"	100 to 131 lbs.	132 to 157 lbs.	158 to 206 lbs.
5' 2"	104 to 135 lbs.	136 to 163 lbs.	164 to 213 lbs.
5' 3"	107 to 140 lbs.	141 to 168 lbs.	169 to 220 lbs.
5' 4"	110 to 144 lbs.	145 to 173 lbs.	174 to 227 lbs.
5' 5"	114 to 149 lbs.	150 to 179 lbs.	180 to 234 lbs.
5' 6"	118 to 154 lbs.	155 to 185 lbs.	186 to 241 lbs.
5' 7"	121 to 158 lbs.	159 to 190 lbs.	191 to 249 lbs.
5' 8"	125 to 163 lbs.	164 to 196 lbs.	197 to 256 lbs.
5' 9"	128 to 168 lbs.	169 to 202 lbs.	203 to 263 lbs.
5' 10"	132 to 173 lbs.	174 to 208 lbs.	209 to 271 lbs.
5' 11"	136 to 178 lbs.	179 to 214 lbs.	215 to 279 lbs.
6' 0"	140 to 183 lbs.	184 to 220 lbs.	221 to 287 lbs.
6' 1"	144 to 188 lbs.	189 to 226 lbs.	227 to 295 lbs.
6' 2"	148 to 193 lbs.	194 to 232 lbs.	233 to 303 lbs.
6' 3"	152 to 199 lbs.	200 to 239 lbs.	240 to 311 lbs.
BMI	**19 to 24**	**25 to 29**	**30 to 39**

DETERMINE YOUR OWN BMI

BODY MASS INDEX (BMI)

BMI is a way to determine whether your weight is healthy or not.
It is a more useful measurement than actual weight.

BMI _____

Underweight: < 18.5   Normal: 18.5 - 25
Overweight: 25 - 30   Obese: 30 <

Weight (lbs)		x 703 =		(A)
Height (in)	x	Height (in)	=	(B)
(A)	÷	(B)	=	BMI

I could go into all the scary facts—and I will in Chapter 2—about how being overweight or obese is linked to diabetes, cancer, heart disease, and even stroke, but what does this really mean to you? Don't get me wrong; I'm sure you care about your long-term health, but it's much easier for you to see your health in smaller, more recognizable, everyday issues. Maybe you wake up tired after what should have been a good night's rest. You find yourself relying on coffee and energy drinks to even get through the day. Your kiddos complain that you no longer have the energy to play with them. Headaches are more frequent, you can't walk up the stairs without losing your breath, not to mention your knee and joint pain. And we won't get you started on the bickering from your husband or wife about your new nighttime habit of snoring. All of these aliments are oh-so-common conditions directly linked to packing on the pounds, or as it is sometimes called, the battle of the bulge. No matter what you call it, how do you solve it?

Before I give you the tools to solve your overweight dilemma, it is incredibly important for you to know *why* you got fat in the first place. Knowing the why makes all the difference.

We live in a toxic world, full of overprocessed foods, containing hidden chemicals and sugars, both natural and artificial, invented by Food Inc. to get you to buy what they are selling. And boy, have we. Humans consume more calories than ever before. On average, men and women consume somewhere between 200 to 400 calories above the recommended intake, daily. While this may seem marginal, 200 calories a day ... what's the big deal? What an extra 200–400 calories a day really means is an extra 1,400–2,800 calories a week. What you may or may not know is that it only takes a deficit or surplus of 3,500 calories to lose or gain one pound. So, in our current example, if you are consuming an extra 200 calories a day, by the end of the month, all things being constant, you will be 2 pounds heavier. Let's take a moment for some quick math: 2 pounds a month = 24 pounds a year. Now, that truly is startling.

IT ONLY TAKES A DEFICIT OR SURPLUS OF 3,500 CALORIES TO LOSE OR GAIN ONE POUND

What's even scarier than how quickly this epidemic can creep up on you, is *how* it has managed to do so in the first place. This epidemic has only been shoved to the forefront of the news cycle since the late '90s. Why is it that our grandparents and their parents didn't face the same issues we have today? Gone are the days of going into our backyard and picking vegetables from our garden for dinner. Today, with all of the hustle and bustle of our busy schedules, Americans often stop for a quick bite to eat at one of the 50,000 fast food restaurant chains conveniently located right around the corner from their home, our kids' soccer practice field, or on the way home from the office. Healthy, home-

Erin Coleman, R.D., L.D., "The Average Calorie Intake by a Human Per Day Versus the Recommendation," sfgate.com, http://healthyeating.sfgate.com/average-calorie-intake-human-per-day-versus-recommendation-1867.html.

cooked meals are an infrequent occurrence due to our busy schedules.

But do you ever wonder how it is these fast food restaurants can keep their food fresh or how they can possibly keep up with the flow of demand? It's actually rather simple, thanks to technology. Fast food chains have found ways to use special additives, preservatives, and—yes, in some instances—chemicals to preserve their foods to mass market to you, the consumer. Even in our fields, farmers are using pesticides, herbicides, and growth hormones to help produce foods that are as large as possible, as quickly as possible, and as cost efficient as possible with no consideration for how those chemicals, hormones, and toxins really affect your body. And this isn't even to speak of the toxins and chemicals we have surrounded ourselves with through the advent of fossil fuels, big pharma, and packaged food companies.

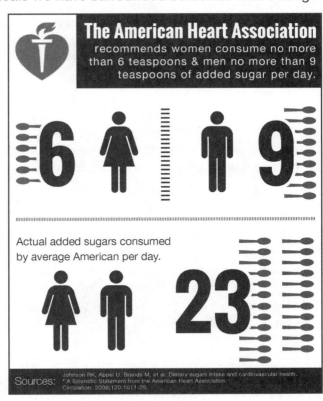

The American Heart Association recommends women consume no more than 6 teaspoons & men no more than 9 teaspoons of added sugar per day.

Actual added sugars consumed by average American per day.

Sources: Johnson RK, Appel LJ, Brands M, et al. Dietary sugars intake and cardiovascular health. A Scientific Statement from the American Heart Association. Circulation. 2009;120:1011-20.

If you have been paying attention to food labels over the years, I am sure you have noticed an influx of disclaimers, clamoring for your attention, that this product contains no artificial ingredients, no high fructose corn syrup, no hydrogenated oils, none of the chemicals that after years and years of use by the general population have given scientists the opportunity to link those same ingredients to cancer in lab rats. The surplus of ingredients used to make food last longer, and therefore available for purchase on grocery store shelves long after their production and transport to the store, is no laughing matter. The surplus of calories we as Americans consume is directly linked to foods that have been highly processed and are now void of any real nutritional value. Of the 600,000 food items on our grocery shelves in America, a staggering 80% have added sugar. Foods are being refined in such a way to produce a drug-like effect in the pleasure and reward center of our brain, making us crave them. What was once fuel for our body, a mechanism to support our output of mental and physical energy, is being modified in such a way that we respond the exact same way drug addicts respond to their choice of poison. It should come as no surprise that foods high in sugar, fat, and salt are the very same triggers of these cravings. By eating these calorically dense foods, we train our body to eat more and more and more. Powered with this knowledge, is it any wonder why some predict that over 95% of Americans will be overweight within 2 decades? In addition to being overweight, it's expected in the same time frame, 1 in every 3 Americans will have diabetes. Knowledge is one of the first steps in solving this epidemic.

In addition to the high-calorie, hormone-latent foods we currently use as staples in our on-the-go diets, as we age we are genetically dispositioned to gain weight. In fact, we face countless issues that actually aid in weight—specifically, fat—gain the older we get. What is known as our metabolic rate, more commonly referred to as our metabolism, slows down. This means our body then requires less calories to sustain our current body composition. In addition, our heart and lung function slows, making the same calorie expenditure previously performed through workouts not as productive. As if that weren't enough, it's not uncommon for us to lose muscle mass as we age, which also reduces the amount of calories we need to eat. Aches and pains

Fed Up, directed by Stephanie Soechtig (2014; RADiUS-TWC, May 2014), Netflix.

pop up more frequently, which reduces our desire to get out and be active. Starting to see a pattern? The odds are stacked against us.

In addition to the why, it's important you understand how to differentiate between the fats you have in your body. Subcutaneous fat, that which you can see on your body and can pinch, is what most people strive to lose. But the most deadly kind of fat is called visceral fat. Visceral fat is the fat stored in and around your organs in your abdominal cavity and actually releases hormones that can even further hinder your weight loss problems.

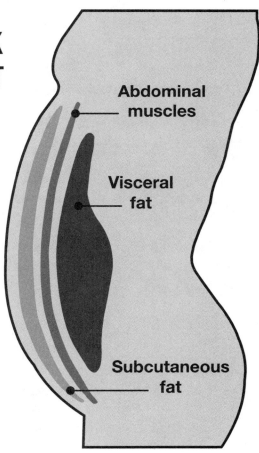

THE INSIDE LOOK @VISCERAL FAT

Abdominal muscles

Visceral fat

Subcutaneous fat

CHAPTER 1: TAKEAWAYS

1. We live in a toxic world.

2. Our foods are overprocessed.

3. Sugar is poisoning our body.

4. Of the 600,000 food items on our grocery shelves in America, a staggering 80% have added sugar.

5. Subcutaneous fat is that which you can see on your body.

6. The most dangerous kind of fat is visceral. Visceral fat is stored in and around your organs.

CHAPTER 2

THE **STRUGGLE** IS **REAL...**
THE **CHALLENGES** OF **OBESITY**

It is of utmost importance you understand the truly destructive —and—in far too many cases, deadly—reasons why you should care about the extra weight you're forced to tote around. Even the most basic of reasons—how we look, how little energy we have, and even the joint injuries and aliments we've sustained all pale in comparison to the cumbersome toll excess fat weighs on your health. Cancer, stroke, diabetes: I really could go on and on. And I will. This chapter serves as a ghostly reminder of what is to come if we can't overcome the adversity Food Inc. has laid before us. No longer can we rely on our government to oversee and encourage the food industry to provide good, wholesome food on our local grocery shelves. My hope is this chapter, be it dark and scary, but necessary, lights a fire inside you that will continue

GET BACK TO THE BASICS OF FOOD, ENSURING YOU CAN FINALLY...

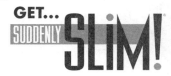

to fuel your desire to create a new relationship with food, one where we get back to the basics of food, ensuring you can finally Get *Suddenly Slim*.

DIABETES – Doctors refer to bodies that lack the ability to produce insulin (type 1), or produce too little or can no longer use it effectively (type 2) as diabetes. Diabetes is often the most discussed result of filling our bodies with toxic, processed, and fat-latent foods. Ironically, as diabetes cases have doubled in the last 30 years, so too has consumption of sugar. In spite of watching what you eat, only buying food that is advertised as low in fat, or reduced fat, you are still faced with an epidemic that haunts 2 out of every 3 Americans.

TRICKING CONSUMERS INTO THINKING THESE FOODS WERE A HEALTHIER WAY OF EATING, THE "LIGHT/REDUCED FAT" REVOLUTION HAD UNFORESEEN CONSEQUENCES.

The surge in consumption is largely due to the McGovern report of 1977, which was deceptively manipulated by the meat, dairy, and other interest-prone food industries. The McGovern report taught the American public to purchase consumables that are lower in fat, cholesterol, and calories. A noble and harmless suggestion by itself, but this only spurred billion-dollar food industries to the creation of a "Light/Reduced Fat" marketing revolution. Tricking consumers into thinking these foods were a healthier way of eating, the "Light/Reduced Fat" revolution had unforeseen consequences. Here is one: the skyrocketing rate of adolescent diabetes, grew from 0 cases in 1980 to an astronomical 57,638 in 2010.

HEART DISEASE – A very general term, heart disease is most often diagnosed when blood vessels that carry blood to the heart begin to harden, narrow, and thus restrict flow. Blood vessels have been pinpointed as one of the casualties of a diet high in sugar and saturated and trans fats that now fill the middle rows of our

Fed Up, directed by Stephanie Soechtig (2014; RADiUS-TWC, May 2014), Netflix.

grocery stores. These fats are hard and not as easy for the body to digest.

HIGH BLOOD PRESSURE – The strength with which blood pushes through your arteries is what is known as blood pressure. High blood pressure is intertwined with being overweight because your body, more specifically your heart, has to pump harder to supply blood to all of your cells. As you can imagine, pushing too hard can weaken your cells, especially in the brain, which when weakened, leak and rupture, causing strokes.

KIDNEY DISEASE – Your kidney's job is to filter toxins and waste, along with unnecessary fluid, out of your blood. In a single day, a healthy kidney filters 200 gallons of blood. As with anything, the harder and more unnecessarily it works, the greater the chance for overuse and, as such, failure.

REPRODUCTIVE ISSUES – Carrying too much fat reduces the chances of not only conceiving, but of carrying a healthy baby to full term. Infertility issues are often caused by the hormonal imbalances associated with obesity. This is not exclusive to women; an overweight father can also affect the woman's chances of getting pregnant due to an insufficient amount or even poor quality of sperm.

SLEEP APNEA – According to the National Heart, Lung, and Blood Institute, an estimated 18 million Americans suffer from sleep apnea, a disorder that is identified by one or more pauses in breath while you sleep. These pauses can last anywhere from just a few seconds to a minute or more until breathing restarts, which is usually accompanied by a snort or choking sound. Episodes of apnea can occur once to one hundred times an hour. The downside to sleep apnea probably goes without saying, but in addition to the loss of oxygen in your blood, it hinders the amount of rest you actually get, reducing your energy levels tremendously.

All of these health issues are lasting consequences of filling our bodies with the wrong foods. Even though Food Inc. would have you believe they have modified unhealthy foods into *light,* or *reduced* and *low-fat* versions, these unnatural laboratory food adjustments have just traded one deadly ingredient for another.

Something else you need to understand that most people don't, is this is not your fault, and you are not alone. In addition to being just one of millions of Americans duped by the food industry, your body produces hormones you have no control over. Years of filling our bodies with both *low-fat,* overprocessed foods, and using artificial sweeteners whenever we can has caused our hunger hormones to lose control. Leptin, the satiety hormone, signals to the brain to inhibit additional calorie consumption. On the opposite end of the spectrum, ghrelin, the hunger hormone, tells your brain you need more. This is yet another hormone affected by years of inadequate nutrition paired with an abundance of just plain bad foods have resulted in decreased sensitivity to leptin. But, ghrelin stays just as strong as it ever was, keeping you seemingly never satisfied.

YEARS OF INADEQUATE NUTRITION PAIRED WITH AN ABUNDANCE OF JUST PLAIN BAD FOODS HAVE RESULTED IN DECREASED SENSITIVITY TO LEPTIN.

It is true that some individuals are genetically susceptible, and even prone to weight gain, while others have these diseases passed down in their genes. But at the end of the day, no matter what you eat, you are on a diet. If you put food in your mouth, you are on a diet. What your diet is comprised of is entirely up to you, and you alone. You have the option to fill your body with things that come branded, prepackaged, likely seen on commercials, or you can allow me to teach you how to make food work in your favor. Good, healthy food doesn't have to taste bad. With a bit of information and a desire to better yourself, preparing food in a healthy way will eventually become second nature. Some say it takes 21 days to form a habit. But, when you're done with this book, I am going to ask you to grant me an extra 9 days and experience how the *Suddenly Slim* Weight Loss Program, can chisel away the fat and create lasting, lifelong eating habits to build a stronger, healthier you.

On any given day, 120 million Americans are on a weight loss program (according to studies published in the Journal of American Medical Association). People will often try more than 5 different ways to lose weight before completely giving up. With more than 50 years in the health, weight loss, and wellness industry, I feel privileged to have helped thousands upon thousands of people lose weight successfully and keep it off with my special weight-loss programs and supplements. In addition to watching substantial life changes in these people I consider family, I continually surround myself with the most renowned doctors, nutritional scientists, and holistic practitioners in the world to keep my products not only up to date, but the best on the market. Additionally, our *Suddenly Slim* Weight Loss Program comes complete with 4 all-natural supplements and a full nutritional menu guide. We have real people, eating real food, and getting real results, losing as much as 1 pound a day. Can you imagine how you would feel in 30 days averaging a loss of even ½ a pound a day?

CHAPTER 2: TAKEAWAYS

1. Being overweight and obese has serious health consequences.

2. With *Suddenly Slim* you can lose up to 1 pound a day.

3. You are no longer alone in your struggle. You will be part of our *Suddenly Slim* community who will help and motivate you along your journey.

4. With *Suddenly Slim*'s menu guide, we have identified exactly which foods will give you the success you seek in weight loss. No more guessing or calorie counting—just wholesome, nutritious foods.

5. *Suddenly Slim* teaches you how to transform your eating patterns and create lasting, lifelong eating habits.

6. *Suddenly Slim*'s line of supplements provide all the nutrient support your body needs to ensure your body gets everything it needs.

CHAPTER 3

CALORIES IN VS. CALORIES OUT

Calories in versus calories out is certainly not a new concept. In fact, it's one you have probably heard before. However, I am are here to tell you, **it is not a reliable tool in your weight loss arsenal** when served at face value. To explain and grasp the concept fully, I would be doing you a disservice if I didn't familiarize you with a few key components of nutrition. The first is that a calorie is defined as the energy needed to raise the temperature of water by one degree. Simplified, a calorie is how much energy resides in food, and in response, how much energy your body will need to produce to use it in its entirety.

Your food is made up of 3 macronutrients: protein, carbohydrates, and fats. Of those, carbs and fats have identified important subcategories.

CARBS: The total carbohydrate content in your food can be made up of carbohydrates, sugars, fiber, or sugar alcohols, all of which determine if the food, as a whole, is classified as a slow-digesting or fast-digesting carbohydrate. You may have heard of this concept before as well, called the GI, or glycemic index. The GI is another tool to help you identify which foods, eaten individually, are actually good for your body. Going a step deeper, the GI classifies foods that will enact a positive digestive response, which is the reason we eat food in the first place, right?

GI | GLYCEMIC INDEX CHART

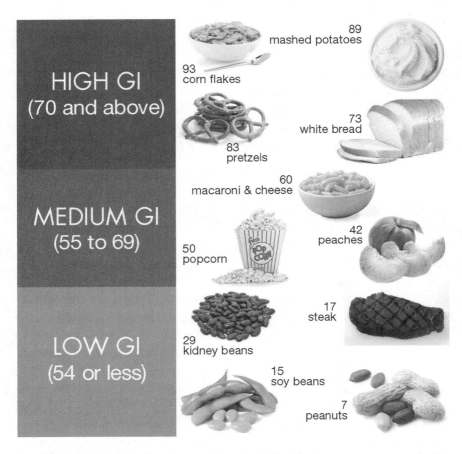

HIGH GI
(70 and above)

89
mashed potatoes

93
corn flakes

73
white bread

83
pretzels

MEDIUM GI
(55 to 69)

60
macaroni & cheese

42
peaches

50
popcorn

LOW GI
(54 or less)

17
steak

29
kidney beans

15
soy beans

7
peanuts

The glycemic index measures the blood glucose response of specific foods from 1 to 100. Foods with high GI numbers are considered to be fast-digesting, while low GI numbers signal that the food is slower to digest. Low GI foods have been proven to have benefits for weight control due to the way they can better control fat-signaling hormones like insulin. Low GI foods also keep you full longer as they are often higher in fiber than foods at the opposite end of the scale.

Glycemic Index, The University of Sydney, last modified October 12, 2015, http://www.glycemicindex.com/

FATS: A confusing concept to some, I want to be sure I am clear—the fats you ingest are not the same as that which you can see and feel. Just because you eat fat doesn't mean you will get fat. In reality, your body can take excess amounts of any macronutrient provided—protein, carbohydrates, or fat—and mold it into subcutaneous or visceral fat. Your body requires fat for cognitive function. Made up of almost 60% fat, your brain needs a constant supply of essential fatty acids to function properly and avoid haze and fog that can flood your mind when malnourished. EFAs are what remains of fats, such as cooking

THE SKINNY ON FATS...

UNSATURATED **FATS** (there are 2 different **kinds...**)

MONOUNSATURATED FAT (good for you)

- avocado
- nuts & nut butters
- olive oil

POLYUNSATURATED FAT (not-so-bad for you)

- salmon
- sunflower seeds
- soybean, sunflower, or corn oil

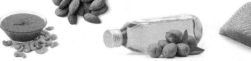

SATURATED **FAT**
(not-so-good for you)

- high fat animal meats
- whole fat dairy
- coconut oil

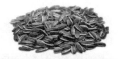

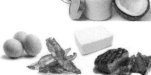

TRANS **FAT**
(bad for you)

- packaged foods
- cookies & donuts
- fried foods

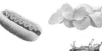

oils, nuts, and avocados, after they have been broken down by the body. Fats can be saturated or unsaturated. Each kind of fat possesses specific properties, and much like a balance of macros, it's important that you also have a balance of fats to take advantage of their properties, which include lowering your bad cholesterol (LDL) levels or being anti inflammatory. With this knowledge, can you see why adding fats into your diet that counteract the buildup of bad (LDL) cholesterol and calm inflammation can aid in weight loss?

So, now that you understand the basics, let me explain why there is a fundamental flaw in the Calories In vs. Calories Out model. All calories are not created equal. A calorie isn't just a calorie anymore. The GI scale was developed to explain just that. When eaten, all foods elicit a different level of response and hormone release, most notable for our conversation, insulin. Insulin, released by your pancreas after eating, is responsible for keeping blood sugar levels from rising too high—hyperglycemia, or dipping too low—hypoglycemia. The release of insulin is used as a means to allow your body to use glucose, what carbohydrates are eventually broken down into, for immediate energy or to store it for later use. When I say store, I mean just that. Insulin takes glucose by the hand (glucose alone cannot pass through cells) in order to move the excess glucose that is not needed immediately for later energy use in the liver. If the liver is full: you guessed it, glucose cozies up in an existing fat cell, or if they are all full, creates a new cell. The peaks and valleys of blood sugar is one very pivotal reason why we gain weight. As I'm sure you can imagine, insulin is better managed in a steady, but low dose versus spikes that prevent your brain from realizing your body is full, and valleys that cause you to get cranky, weak, and overconsume at the first opportunity. This is why we advise you on how frequently to eat in the *Suddenly Slim* Menu Guide, keeping your blood sugar as level as possible with the right kinds of food.

Insulin is often thought of as the perpetuator of weight gain, the bad guy everyone can point their finger at, especially so when you throw diabetes into the mix, but insulin is necessary to our body's function. Without insulin, we wouldn't be able to utilize carbohydrates for energy, which is crucial to our survival. It wasn't until Food Inc. redesigned the basic, natural makeup of our food that we had real, lasting, and devastating issues centered on insulin. Food Inc.'s role is why our grandparents and their parents didn't deal with the same obesity epidemic we have been served. Instead of providing our bodies with fibrous, leafy vegetables and lean cuts of meat, we are shoveling down foods that were invented in laboratories so they could withstand a long shelf life and washing down that "meal" with a sugary beverage. Energy balance, a calorie in vs. calories out, does not work in the society in which we live today, this world that offers highly-processed, genetically modified, and refined foods as acceptable food staples. While that barely scratched the surface, I trust that when I say, a calorie isn't a calorie, we are all on the same page.

I want to leave you with this nugget: you need calories to survive. Everyone has a BMR, basal metabolic rate, which identifies just how many calories (for the most part) a healthy, individual requires to maintain vital functions inside the body and their current body composition at rest. At rest literally means if a 150 pound, 5'5", 35-year-old woman were to hypothetically lay in bed all day, doing absolutely nothing, she would need around 1,400 calories to maintain her current composition. BMR is a scientific calculation that takes into considerations your age, height, weight, and sex. To find how many calories you need daily, you add a specific amount of calories to your BMR, adjusting for your activity level, be it sedentary, active, or very active. Something extremely important to note, with all of the fad and starvation diets that are prevalent today is that your metabolic rate could differ from the calculation. Years of yo-yo dieting, overexercising, and starvation diets can do, in some cases, irreparable damage to your metabolism. Years of starving yourself can cause your body to adapt to the amount of calories you give it and allow your body to substantially lower the amount of calories it requires for your BMR. Working out 2 and 3 times a day, for hours at a time, as you've seen on countless television shows, causes tremendous initial weight loss, yes. But eventually, your body wises up to your antics. It sees through your

THE HUMAN BODY IS AN INCREDIBLY SMART ORGANISM THAT DEVOTES 100% OF ITS ATTENTION TO NOT ONLY PROTECTING, BUT PRESERVING ITSELF.

methods of shocking it into change and adapts accordingly. It goes into starvation mode and prevents fat loss, or even worse, burns muscle and continues to hold fat captive, a prisoner, for as long as possible as it settles in for the long haul. You have to give credit where credit is due: the human body is an incredibly smart organism that devotes 100% of its attention to not only protecting, but preserving itself.

For these very specific reasons, reasons that most people don't even know were possible, I created the *Suddenly Slim* Menu Guide, which, rather than counting calories until you're blue in the face, identifies food your body needs to start anew, foods that, within reason, you could eat unlimited amounts of and still shed fat. I'm happy to welcome you to the *Get Suddenly Slim* Weight Loss Program, where you are no longer in the dark. Now you know. But are you excited to learn more? Just wait: I will arm you with everything you need to know and more to lose weight and keep it off forever.

CHAPTER 3: TAKEAWAYS

1. The types of food you eat are just as important as calories in vs. calories out. Stick to nonprocessed and unrefined foods.

2. Even if you lose some fat, exercising more doesn't cure the weight problem. You can't outwork a bad diet.

3. We eat food for energy. If you don't consume the right foods, you won't get the right energy.

4. You need a healthy mix of fats, carbs, and protein to create a balanced diet.

5. There are foods you can eat virtually unlimited amounts of and still lose fat.

6. Your diet needs to be high in fiber to lower the digestion rate of foods, keep you full, and prevent constipation.

CHAPTER 4

WATER:
THE **MIRACLE** NUTRIENT

Water is an essential nutrient to keep your body functioning properly. Water is used as a temperature regulator, prevents and alleviates joint pains, and flushes out toxins from the body. Most people know that we need water to survive, but do you know why it is so important?

The body is made up of 70% water, and in order to maintain that balance, you need to drink as much as you release through perspiration, urination, and exhalation. Yes, every time we breathe, especially while we sleep in the comfort of our air-conditioned homes, we exhale water vapor. A tell-tale sign of dehydration comes in the form of bad breath. Water is required in the production of saliva, which contains antibacterial properties. After a full night of sleep, and often losing more than a pound of water, your body has also slowed production of saliva, which gives bacteria free reign. Try to drink a big glass of water as soon as you wake up to help offset dehydration. In addition to combating dehydration, drinking water first thing in the morning allows water to help flush the colon and cause a bowl movement, further cleansing your body of toxins and preventing constipation.

Coming in only after our beloved soft drinks, bottled water is the second most popular beverage in the US. While the battle of bottled water versus tap water rages on, I personally wish the conversation would shift from which water to MORE water. One might think water being the second most popular beverage suggests that we drink enough, but that couldn't be further from the truth.

Most people wait until they feel the scratchy craving in their throat before they reach for a drink, but thirst is often one of the last signs of dehydration. Dehydration symptoms include everything from a dry, sticky mouth to constipation, headaches, dizziness or lightheadedness. Less than optimal fluid in your system can also cause dry skin and even fatigue, making it crucial for weight loss and health in general. Proactively drink water, and sip it throughout the day, regardless of your thirst level.

Water helps quell cravings, especially those for sweets, which your brain and body know are abundant in glucose. Water is dependent in the release of energy stores, such as glycogen (formerly glucose from broken down carbohydrates), and without it, your body simply can't pull it from your fat cells or convert it into glucose to burn it as fuel. So when water isn't readily available, your body then employs anything it can in its search for energy, making way for those pesky cravings.

> **PROACTIVELY DRINK WATER, AND SIP IT THROUGHOUT THE DAY, REGARDLESS OF YOUR THIRST LEVEL.**

Dehydration can also be caused by our consumption of common beverages like coffee, tea, and alcohol, all of which are mild diuretics, and flush liquids out of the body. With our sugar consumption causing dipping energy levels, most of us turn to coffee, which actually further complicates the issue. And to make matters worse, without proper hydration, you can't think as clearly. I bet your midday crash is beginning to make a bit more sense, right?

Another all-too-common sign of dehydration are frequent

headaches. Your brain rests in a sack of fluid that keeps it in place, albeit floating. Dehydration depletes the level of fluid in your sack, and headaches often occur because your brain bumps into your skull. Next time a headache strikes, reach for the water before you pop an Advil or Aleve. Masking the symptoms with pain relievers might provide immediate relief, but if you're dehydrated, water will provide lasting relief.

For most people, getting 6-8 glasses a day is enough, but if you want to be sure you are spot on, I recommend my very specific formula for water consumption. Take your weight, cut that number in half and add 8. This is the number, in ounces, you should drink daily. If you need to lose more than 25 pounds, add an additional 8 ounces of water to your daily intake for every 25 pounds that you want to lose. So if you weigh 150 pounds, use the formula of 150/2+8 so that you consume 83 ounces of water, roughly 2/3 of a gallon, every single day to replenish what your body will use.

> **TAKE YOUR WEIGHT, CUT THAT NUMBER IN HALF AND ADD 8. THIS IS THE NUMBER, IN OUNCES, YOU SHOULD DRINK DAILY.**

Because I don't advise you wait for symptoms, there are 2 simple ways to tell if you are dehydrated.

The Skin Test: Pinch the skin at the top of your hand (reverse your palm) and let go. If your skin goes back immediately, you are likely sufficiently hydrated. If it noticeably takes more than a second or 2, chances are you should get some water in that body!

The Urine Test: If you are well hydrated, your urine should be clear, maybe a tiny hue of yellow. But the darker it gets, the less hydrated you are. If its green, you are either doomed or have one of those toilet bowl cleansers and need to try again later!

TIPS FOR GETTING IN MORE WATER:

- Invest in a BPA-free water bottle and make a point to bring it with you everywhere you can.

- Spice up your water with cucumbers and or lemons.

- Fill your plate with produce. Foods like fruits and veggies are loaded in water. As an example, tomatoes and watermelons are more than 90% water!

- While ice water burns more calories in the digestive process than room temperature water, it can sometimes be hard to drink. It is more important to get in the water than take advantage of its calorie-burning qualities.

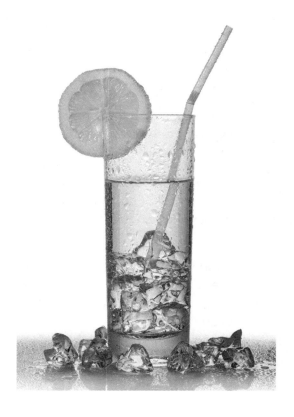

CHAPTER 4: TAKEAWAYS

1. Your body is made up of 70% water.

2. Most people suffer from dehydration.

3. To maximize weight loss: take your body weight, divide it in half and add 8 to this number. This is the number, in ounces, of water you should drink daily.

4. More often than not, hunger pains are actually your body wanting water, not food.

5. Fruits and veggies are loaded in water. Some are as much as 90% water!

6. Cold water burns more calories because your body has to convert it to room temperature.

CHAPTER 5

FOODSTUFF: THE **GOOD**

Every day we wake up, we are presented with the opportunity to start our day fresh, break our fast with a wholesome, nutritious meal. Plain and simple, this chapter will guide you through what foods will fuel your success in weight loss, as well as maintenance once you achieve your desired weight.

As you may recall from Chapter 3, we discussed the 3 macronutrients that make up calories: proteins (4 calories per gram), carbohydrates (4 calories per gram), and fats (9 calories per gram).

The body needs BCAAs, branch-chain amino acids, to build, repair, and maintain muscle—20 different amino acids to be exact. Amino acids are the building blocks of protein. Each amino acid plays host to a number of different metabolic functions including the breakdown of fat to be regulated as energy, repairing damaged tissue, calcium absorption, and much more. Your body can produce 11 of these, and the other 9, named essential amino acids, have to be supplemented through the foodstuff in your diet. This is why it is so important to ensure you have a well-balanced diet, full of high-quality, complete, lean proteins. A complete protein is one that contains all 9 essential amino acids the body cannot produce.

Proteins can come from animals in the form of meat, including red meat, poultry, and fish. Animals can also provide proteins in the form of dairy (cheese, milk), soy, and eggs. Vegan and vegetarian protein options also extend to produce such as beans, nuts, and seeds, as well as lentils. While the last 3 food sources—nuts, seeds, and lentils—represent food that contain high percentages of protein, they are actually classified as a fat or carbohydrate and not a complete protein. That is not to say you couldn't mix and match food to create a meal that is a complete protein. For example, beans and rice served separately are incomplete, but served together, they make up all 9 essential amino acids. The classification of macronutrient rests on the percentage of their macronutrient breakdown. If the majority of their calories come from protein, they are a protein. And the same holds true for fats and carbohydrates.

Every person is different, and as such, so too are their protein requirements. Some can make do with the minimum recommended amount of protein, which is .36 grams per pound of body weight. In our 150 pound female example, that would be about 55 grams a day. It should be noted, this amount is purely to prevent protein deficiency and all 55 grams would be used daily in protein turnover. This means others who are more active and exercise frequently need much more protein to prevent catabolization, your body burning your muscles. Anywhere from .5 grams per pound of body weight for someone mildly active, about 75 grams a day. Someone who lifts weights routinely or works in a very physical job should supplement their diet with even more protein, like 1–1.2 grams per pound of body weight (150–180 grams in the same example). Note: BCAAs are the secret here again to avoid catabolism.

Now, as I touched on earlier, it's important you keep your protein sources lean. Yes, you can get 26 grams of protein from your beloved Big Mac, but at what cost? Each Big Mac has a whopping 33 grams of fat which is ½ of your daily recommended value.

SUDDENLY SLIM

LEAN PROTEINS

Up to 8 oz. of lean meat, fish, or poultry, skin removed.

BODY FX® SHAKES

DAIRY & EGGS
- Eggs (2 any style)
- Low-Fat Cottage or
  Ricotta Cheese (1/2 cup)
- Low-Fat Yogurt (1 cup)
- Skim Milk (8 oz)

FISH
- All Fresh Fish
- Tuna (water packed)

MEAT
- Beef or Lamb (lean)
- Ham (center cuts only)
- Veal (in moderation)
- Venison, Bison, Buffalo

POULTRY
- Chicken (breast)
- Turkey (breast)

SOUPS
- Bean Soup
- Vegetable Soup

VEGETARIAN
- Lentils (any kind)
- Beans (any kind)
- Tofu
- Tempeh

It's also important to mention that most protein elicits a minimal glucose response, meaning proteins are rather low on the GI. If you combine protein with every meal, it has the potential to lower the entire meal's GI value. Much like carbohydrates, protein also has options that are slow and fast digesting. Fast-digesting proteins are those which are already in liquid form, such as egg

EVERYONE CAN AND SHOULD UTILIZE SLOW-DIGESTING, UNPROCESSED, HIGH-FIBER CARBOHYDRATES SUCH AS VEGETABLES, BEANS, BROWN RICE, QUINOA, AND SPROUT BREADS, WHICH WILL HELP YOU STAY FULL, PREVENT SUGAR CRAVINGS, AND HELP KEEP YOU ON TRACK.

whites (the yolk, high in fat, slows down digestion) and whey protein powders. Slower-digesting proteins are typically solid, like meats, as well as casein protein powder, which was intentionally incorporated into *Suddenly Slim*'s Body FX® meal replacement protein shake. The more slowly the protein digests, the steadier your blood glucose levels remain.

As you may recall, carbohydrates, also called carbs, are essential to your body's metabolism. Required by the body to produce energy, both immediately and to store for later use in the form of glucose, a minimum intake of 130 grams of carbs has been established by the American Dietetic Association. In addition to needing carbs for energy, this minimum has been set to provide enough glucose for the brain to perform at optimal levels.

It's important you fuel your carbohydrate requirements with high-fiber, slow-digesting carbs, especially while focusing on losing weight. Strategically eating high-fiber vegetables and carbs that are slower-digesting like whole grain breads, brown rice, and even fruit, allow not only for steady blood sugar levels, but also an overall feeling of being "full," or what is known as satiety.

To summarize, carbs are not something you should fear, but learn about and pay close attention to in order to maximize your weight loss potential. It's the most variable macronutrient and the amount necessary differs from person to person, depending on your body type and daily activity level. Everyone can and should utilize slow-digesting, unprocessed, high-fiber carbohydrates such as vegetables, beans, brown rice, quinoa, and sprout breads, which will help you stay full, prevent sugar cravings, and help keep you on track. Keep in mind, carbs are needed by most people only to replenish the glucose lost in day-to-day activity. If we can't immediately utilize the carbs we ingest, we will store them. With that said, one of the best habits to kick is our nightly routine of plopping down on the couch in front of the TV to devour a hearty, carb-filled dinner. To optimize fat loss, steer clear of carbs at least 4 hours before bed. Generally speaking, you should be sure your last snack or meal is low in carbs and before 6 PM to maximum results.

SUPPLEMENT YOUR DIET WITH FATS THAT ARE MOSTLY UNSATURATED, HIGH IN OMEGA 3, 6, AND 9, FOUND IN NUTS, EGG YOLKS, AVOCADOS, WALNUTS, PISTACHIOS, ALMONDS, AND FATTIER FISH LIKE SALMON.

Our last, often misunderstood, macronutrient is fat. Fats help keep your blood sugar steady and prevent a glucose spikes as all varieties are slow-digesting food.

In addition to your blood glucose levels, your carb intake and your fat intake should always be directly proportionate to one another. At times when your carbohydrates are high, your fats should be lower and vice versa. Most people who get overweight in the first place experience optimal fat loss on diets in which calories are higher from fats than from carbs. This occurs because those individuals who have a tendency to gain weight easily or those who are already overweight have a higher sensitivity to insulin than someone who is at their ideal weight. If you remember, insulin releases its highest doses in conjunction with the digestion of carbohydrates that are high on the GI. Fats, along with protein, come in very low on the GI scale. This is why many people have huge success with low-carb diets. However, I want to stress that it's important you don't cut carbs out from your diet completely. If you follow a low-carb diet, you will likely get results, and relatively quickly, but you will also gain the weight back, often plus additional weight once carbs are reintroduced to your diet. Low carb diets are not long-term dieting options.

You might have noticed that fats have a higher caloric value per gram. This isn't a bad thing, but it's definitely something you should consider and take care not to overeat. Fats being 2 times as calorically dense as both protein and carbs are one way people get themselves into trouble. You can overeat healthy foods, especially fats, and put on excess weight because of it.

Like carbs, it's important for you to be able to differentiate between the good and the bad varieties to achieve a balanced diet. As I mentioned, eating fat is crucial for your cognitive function. Supplement your diet with fats that are mostly unsaturated, high in Omega 3, 6, and 9, found in nuts, egg yolks, avocados, walnuts, pistachios, almonds, and fattier fish like salmon. Fat intake is important to the longevity of your health and the overall success of your diet.

CHAPTER 5: TAKEAWAYS

1. Consume 6-8 ounces of lean protein at every meal.

2. Keep your carbs slow-digesting or complex throughout the day. No carbs at least 4 hours before bed.

3. Eat high quality fats to lose fat like unsaturated fats, high in Omega 3, 6, and 9.

4. The *Suddenly Slim* Menu Guide identifies all of the fats you should eat.

5. To lower the GI load of a meal, each meal should have a lean protein, a complex carbohydrate, and healthy fat foods incorporated into it.

6. To manage your weight loss, keep your meals small but satisfying, and incorporate foods from the *Suddenly Slim* menu.

CHAPTER 6

FOODSTUFF: THE **BAD**

With the abundant options and strategic placement of food on today's shelves, it really is no wonder we are where we are. Supermarkets pay incredible attention to food merchandising. They often have nationwide policies not just for branding the stores to look alike, but to maximize your visit by putting the foods you want front and center. The cheapest, but also best tasting, foods are placed at eye level. Store brands or inexpensive foods are often placed at the eye level of an adult and snacks advertised on Nickelodeon and Disney Channels are positioned at our children's eye level. Higher quality, and thus more expensive foods, are often at the top of the shelf, elevating their status (top-shelf) and also staying just out of reach for people who are on a budget. It's a tricky game and one they are winning.

Playing on the wants and desires of consumers, they do not promote (either by placement or price) items that are purchased often and weekly by most consumers. They allow bad foods to follow you around the store, and even at the checkout hoping you will finally give in if you haven't already. One very important tactic I teach is to go to the store with a list, and only after having a snack, meal, or a Body FX® shake. It helps you get in and get out not only faster with only the items you need, but will save you money week after week as you resist the urge to splurge on items you didn't intend to buy in the first place.

Having discussed the macronutrients your body needs and recommended specific examples of high-quality foods within each category, it's important I pinpoint foods that hinder your success. After reading this chapter, you will be able to identify exactly which foods, even if the packaging or branding of the item suggest otherwise, will not benefit your body or your goals.

PROTEIN: Even though a meat, or food, is high in protein, it does not make it a healthy option. Moreover, it does not mean it will help you in your weight loss journey. A considerable amount of red meat should be completely disregarded if not forever, for the most part, while you are trying to lose weight. In red meat, you can clearly see its fat content, or as the industry refers to it, marbling, which gives steak its flavor. The fat is white or off-white in color, often around the edges, as well as intermingled inside the meat itself. Just looking at the offering can alert you to something that is higher in fat. It is, however, a bit harder to see in chicken and turkey. Pay attention to labels, but ground varieties like 80/20, 85/15 should be avoided as one serving of ground beef has 15g of fat! Even scarier, most restaurants don't even use 80/20 but something fattier!

AVOID: Cuts of meat higher in fat than 10 grams including: red meat categorized as prime or choice, and those classified as brisket, ribs, or porterhouse. Check labels, which are found on the underside of most meat packages.

CHECK LABELS WHICH ARE FOUND ON THE UNDERSIDE OF MOST MEAT PACKAGES.

Chicken and turkey are frequently staples of a weight loss diet; however, that doesn't mean all cuts are free reign. Among poultry options—thighs, wings, drumsticks, and like red meat—any ground meat that has more fat than 90/10 is of utmost importance to avoid.

Almost all fish are excellent options. While they are not all what most consider to be low fat, their fat is high quality and fat that you should be consuming. It is worth noting you should eliminate the consumption of fish that are high in mercury and traditional bottom feeders. The FDA warns not to eat: tilefish, swordfish, shark, and king mackerel, but you can safely eat up to 12 ounces a week of fish that are low in mercury like tuna (canned, fresh/frozen), salmon, and orange roughy, to name a few. For the healthiest options among the acceptable fish, try to source wild caught versus farm raised.

As for vegetarian protein options, check the labels to be sure that you aren't taking in too much carbohydrate or fat to make up your minimum protein requirements. Body FX®, *Suddenly Slim*'s meal replacement protein shake, is perfect for people who do not eat meat.

Thanks to the glycemic index, it's relatively easy to identify the carbohydrates to avoid: anything refined, with added or artificial sugar, white breads and pastas, potatoes, fruit juice—and I think it goes without saying—candy. Food additives are abundant in the grocery store, so it's especially important you learn how to read food labels. Food options that note low fat, are often created by stripping some of the fat and replacing it with sugar so it still tastes good.

Also on labels, you will find sodium content, which is important to pay attention to as excessive consumption can lead to a host of complications and even major medical problems. The recommended intake is 1,500 mg a day, with the today's average diet being more than twice that.

Trans fats, which raise your cholesterol and contribute to clogging of the arteries, should be avoided all together. Saturated fats, which include animal fat, can be consumed in moderation, but no more than 7% of your daily intake. When trying to avoid these fats, think of anything that is fried: French fries, doughnuts, fried chicken, pizza crusts, creamer, and margarine.

DIRTY DOZEN

The Environmental Working Group has identified foods, aptly named The Dirty Dozen, which, if at all possible, should only be purchased organically due to the amount of pesticides used in the farming of this produce. Also identified are produce, called the clean fifteen, which rank among the lowest in pesticides.

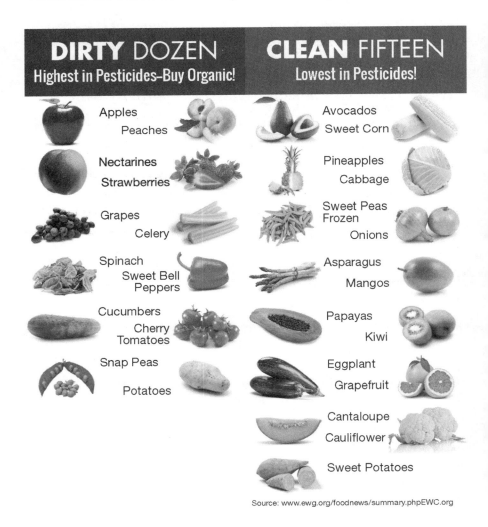

DIRTY DOZEN
Highest in Pesticides-Buy Organic!

CLEAN FIFTEEN
Lowest in Pesticides!

Dirty Dozen	Clean Fifteen
Apples	Avocados
Peaches	Sweet Corn
Nectarines	Pineapples
Strawberries	Cabbage
Grapes	Sweet Peas Frozen
Celery	Onions
Spinach	Asparagus
Sweet Bell Peppers	Mangos
Cucumbers	Papayas
Cherry Tomatoes	Kiwi
Snap Peas	Eggplant
Potatoes	Grapefruit
	Cantaloupe
	Cauliflower
	Sweet Potatoes

Source: www.ewg.org/foodnews/summary.phpEWC.org

Today, 90% of crops have been genetically modified, and almost everything is contaminated with some level of pesticides. To save on the costs of doing business, animals are caged, often never setting foot in an open pasture. Try to frequent farmers markets that can pay closer attention to what they are producing and use less pesticides. Stick to foods that are fresh, and if your budget allows, organic and free range.

> TRY TO FREQUENT FARMERS MARKETS THAT CAN PAY CLOSER ATTENTION TO WHAT THEY ARE PRODUCING AND USE LESS PESTICIDES. STICK TO FOODS THAT ARE FRESH, AND IF YOUR BUDGET ALLOWS, ORGANIC AND FREE RANGE.

It's important we recognize the poor food options that will only hinder our results. In addition to no longer purchasing these products, something we can do right now is audit our pantry and fridge to ensure foods that tempt us are removed from the house. Out of sight, out of mind!

CHAPTER 6: TAKEAWAYS

1. Be aware of food additives and avoid eating foods containing them. Some of the most common are food coloring and high fructose corn syrup.

2. Just because it's made from fruit doesn't make it healthy. Juices are loaded with sugar but come without the fiber from the fruit in natural form, so do not drink fruit juice!

3. Buy organic or local farmers market produce.

4. Avoid meats higher than 10 grams in fat.

5. Food labels can be deceiving. As a general rule, the shorter the ingredient list, the fresher the food.

6. Watch out for cheap, bad foods and avoid having them around to tempt you. Conduct an audit of your food supply today!

CHAPTER 7

FOODSTUFF:
THE **UGLY**

Processed and refined foods need to be eliminated from your diet. This is the first and most important action you can do to begin seeing the changes in your body you want, to restore your energy, and most importantly, to improve your health. Think the fresher the better.

As I stated before, processed and refined foods have been stripped of most of their health benefits and are now void of any real nutritional value. Their carbohydrate content is high in sugar and abundant in artificial ingredients masterfully crafted in labs to assist with flavor. Their fat content is loaded with trans fats as the need to fry virtually everything runs rampant.

> **THE BEST WAY TO CONTROL YOUR WEIGHT LOSS RESULTS IS TO CONTROL WHAT YOU PUT IN YOUR BODY.**

The best way to control your weight loss results is to control what you put in your body. Eliminating fast food entirely will give you the control over your diet you've been lacking. Planning ahead will do wonders for you and your physique.

Certain meats should not only be avoided, but eliminated entirely from your diet. Bacon, sausage, and hot dogs along with deli meats and cold cuts are high in cholesterol and saturated fats. In addition these *"let's just combine what's left over"* meats contain a lot of nitrates, which can be linked to cancer associated with the bladder, esophagus, stomach, and even your brain.

IN ANTICIPATION OF FOOD YOUR BODY STILL RELEASES INSULIN. WHEN IT DOESN'T GET ANY SUGAR, IT RESORTS TO CRAVINGS THAT WILL PLAGUE YOU UNTIL YOU GIVE IN.

Kick sodas to the curb, and in a hurry. Just one 12 ounce coke has 8-10 teaspoons of sugar, which is more sugar than the daily recommended value. Diet sodas, while calorie free, still play tricks on your hormones and body. In anticipation of food your body still releases insulin. When it doesn't get any sugar, it resorts to cravings that will plague you until you give in. People who drink diet sodas put on three times as much belly fat as people who abstain from chemical-filled diet drinks.

MSG is one of the most common, naturally occurring, non essential amino acids. However, it's been cultivated and carefully crafted by the food industry to enrich the taste of food and enhance flavor. While it has been cleared by the FDA and recognized as safe, overconsumption can cause headaches and overall feelings of discomfort. MSG is just one example of the many food additives plaguing our everyday food.

White flour and bread didn't start that way. In fact, white flour actually began life as good, wholesome whole grains! This might make you think there is something healthy to it, but the manufacturers remove the shell, and with it all nutritional value, leaving it yellow or gray in color. Knowing you wouldn't dream of purchasing yellow or gray bread, they add a bleaching ingredient called calcium peroxide to produce the white hue we know and love. Any nutritional value that hadn't already been destroyed can't make it through the bleaching process without being completely denatured. Try not to use the color of the bread as the determining factor for which bread you should buy. With the recent interest in whole grains, companies continue to use white bread processes but add in molasses to create that whole-grain hue. Make sure you pay attention to labels. True whole-grain breads will state 100% whole grain or 100% whole wheat on the package.

Sea salt is derived from evaporating ocean water or salted lake water with little processing. This process leaves behind beneficial minerals. While consuming at, or less than, the daily recommended levels of sodium daily is fine, going above the recommended value, or substituting the healthy option of sea salt for regular table salt, or worse, for processed MSG varieties often found in processed foods, you risk your chances for heart issues and high blood pressure.

Limiting your intake of sugar is the most substantial action we can take in the battle of the bulge. While it will no doubt be difficult to go against our brainwashed hormones and circumvent the sugar system, you will thank me rather quickly. First, you feel energized to take on the day, and possibly even more, when you realize how much money you are saving cutting out all the needless extras like soda and sweets. Sugar is addictive. Study after study reaffirms that once you start consuming these foods, it is just as hard to quit as it would be for an addict to quit his drug of choice. To make matters worse, this food is all around us. An alcoholic can abstain from going into a bar, or even into a restaurant that serves liquor, but no one realistically expects you to go the rest of your life without enjoying a meal out with your family. In fact, on page 85 I will tell you all my weight loss success tips. You are forced to face your addiction head on, everywhere

SUGAR MAKES YOU FAT —PLAIN AND SIMPLE.

you go. Every. Single. Day. Sugar depletes the amount of zinc we have in our body which can dull your sense of taste, requiring an even larger dose, further compounding the problem! Sugar negatively impacts your immune system, has substantial and undeniable links to behavioral disorders, and promotes the theft of calcium from your bones to counteract its acidity level. Sugar makes you fat—plain and simple. The food industry has infiltrated our bodies with sugar at every possible meal. Breakfast: here, start your day off with a glass of sugar—oops, I mean orange juice. Lunch? Swing by McDonald's and enjoy a burger, fries, and a coke. Your 3 PM crash can be fueled with more coffee, sweetened with sugar and cream, of course. This not even taking into consideration the snacking that ensues as we sit on our couch after a long, taxing day sitting down all day at work. We reward ourselves because we work so hard, but we are not dogs. We should not reward ourselves with food!

This all may sound a bit daunting and more than you can tackle on your own, but you are not alone. Our program, which I outline in the next 2 chapters, will take you from exactly where you are and turn your life around. Literally, the changes you will experience with *Suddenly Slim* will affect your entire life. Beyond our program, our ever-growing community will help motivate, encourage, and cheer you on.

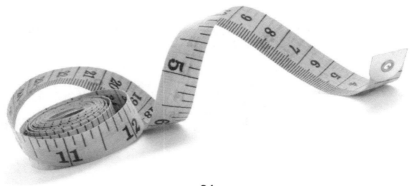

CHAPTER 7: TAKEAWAYS

1. Nutrition has been processed out of most of the food on grocery store shelves.

2. Foods can be as addictive as drugs. Studies have shown that food addicts' brain receptors act similar to those of drug addicts.

3. Manufacturers hide sugar in food.

4. Stop drinking sodas!

5. Limit sodium consumption, instead use sea salt to season your food.

6. Make a conscious decision to eliminate sugar from your diet wherever possible and stick to it!

CHAPTER 8

THE **ANSWER:**
GET... *SUDDENLY SLIM*®

We have arrived to what I consider to be the most exciting and important chapter of this book, the answer for which you have been searching: the weight loss solution for everybody, the program that will stop the struggle and help people physically change their lives, once and for all. Everything you've read up until now have been facts, statistics, and information about what foods are bad, which are good, and even how we, as a nation, got into this mess. Incredibly important knowledge, this information will carry you through your weight-loss journey.

> **THINK OF ME AS YOUR VERY OWN NUTRITIONAL COACH.**

But now, I'm sure you are wondering, how do I condense all of this information and *Get Suddenly Slim*? Don't worry, I have done the work for you. Think of me as your very own nutritional coach.

The answer to your weight-loss woes is called The *Suddenly Slim* Weight Loss Program. *Suddenly Slim* will help you lose weight and reshape your body. Whether you have unwanted pounds, excess body fat, or excess inches—*Suddenly Slim* is your weight loss solution.

The *Suddenly Slim* **Weight Loss Program**:

- Helps curb appetite*
- Helps reduce belly fat*
- Supports fat burning*
- Increases energy*

Plus, helps cleanse the inner body and colon*

Suddenly Slim is comprised of 4 powerful products, a program and menu guide, and is conveniently packaged into 3 affordable programs. Each program is designed to provide inner body cleansing, detoxification, and fat burning properties to achieve the weight loss results you desire.

Before I go over the program distinctions, I want to get down to the basics and introduce you to the lineup of *Suddenly Slim* products that will change your life. Truly, I mean that. Before reading any further, take a look at these *Real People*, who have achieved *Real Results* with my *Suddenly Slim* Weight Loss Program on page 88. Go ahead, I'll wait.

Now that you've seen what I mean when I say "change your life," let me explain the purpose and importance of each product in my *Suddenly Slim* Weight Loss Programs.

My weight loss programs have a foundation that begins with cleansing and detoxifying the body, first and foremost. The cornerstone of a successful weight loss program rests within your body's ability to absorb and process food as it should, which is necessary for successful weight loss and optimal wellness.

RENEÚ® is a botanical formula that delivers nearly 50 herbs to help cleanse and detoxify the inner body and colon. It was specifically formulated to include nutraceuticals that help promote regularity. After years of filling our bodies with toxins and chemicals that pose harm to its ability to function at full capacity, cleansing and detoxifying is the first and most crucial element in the *Suddenly Slim* Weight Loss Program. Ridding your body of literal buildup allows your body to absorb the nutrients from the foods we eat.

*These statements have not been evaluated by the Food and Drug Administration.
This product is not intended to diagnose, treat, cure, or prevent disease.
†When used in conjunction with the Suddenly Slim Program | Menu Guide, which includes diet and exercise.

If you have never cleansed or detoxified, you should know that this will increase your bowl movements. It's important for your body to excrete everything it doesn't digest on a regular basis. Infrequency and irregular bowl movements are a red flag that your body is in desperate need of a cleanse.

Toxins aren't just in the food we eat. They are in the air we breathe, the household products we use to clean our homes, and everywhere we step. Living life on earth without some degree of toxic buildup is, in this day and age, impossible. Cleansing and detoxifying free radicals, toxins, and chemicals from our body will energize our cells and prevent further cellular damage. Cleansing and detoxification is necessary because the systems our body has built in to do that itself are overwhelmed and either no longer function at full capacity or, in many cases, at all due to the influx of pollutants we endure today. There is no escaping toxins. We can only proactively ensure we address these issues often and frequently to achieve optimal health. The cornerstone of my weight loss programs, Reneú® is available in all 3 of my Weight Loss Programs: Boost, Accelerate, and Transformation.

XANOLEAN™ SUPREME contains ingredients that will help reduce your appetite and increase your energy. It is important to feel like yourself while you are on any diet, and energy levels play a big role in the big picture of your success in weight loss. Specific ingredients in the XanoLean™ Supreme formula have also been shown to enhance a natural occurring hormone called dopamine that conveniently signals your body to stop eating. In addition, XanoLean™ Supreme acts as what is commonly referred to as a fat burner. Through advanced thermogenesis, which is the production of heat, your body forces fat

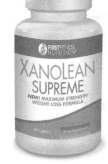

cells to release their grip on fat, which is then transported through the blood for uptake into the muscles to be used as fuel. Using fat for fuel eliminates the fat from your body. XanoLean™ Supreme is incorporated into all three of my Weight Loss Programs: Boost, Accelerate, and Transformation.

BODY FX® is a scientifically formulated, time-released, nutritional meal replacement protein shake. Available in 2 flavors, Tropical Cremé or Chocolate Paradise, it's not only delicious, but has a balanced macronutrient ratio giving your body what it needs. Fifty percent low glycemic carbohydrates, thirty percent protein, and twenty percent fat, we've designed this perfect meal replacement protein shake as an ideal substitute for breakfast, lunch, and dinner. The perfect meal, Body FX® contains vitamins and minerals your body needs, while satisfying your hunger to prevent overeating. A blend of whey and casein protein, Body FX® digests and releases nutrients both quickly, as a result of the whey, and over an extended period of time, thanks to the casein. This dynamic product keeps you full longer and helps stabilize your blood sugar level. I strategically sweetened Body FX® with pure crystalline fructose, which has a GI response (22) considerably lower than traditional carbohydrates. Pure crystalline fructose is classified by the FDA as sugar because of its use as

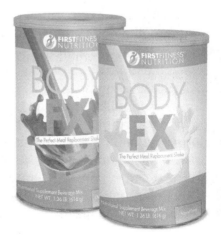

a sweetener, but it does not cause the same blood sugar spike most carbohydrates create. It also contains 3 grams of fiber, which work to further slow the GI response down to that of a traditional protein. The Accelerate Weight Loss Program offers your choice of one flavor of Body FX® and both flavors are available in my Transformation Weight Loss Program.

TRIMBOLIC®, my fat and cellulite fighter, is a dynamic formula of key nutrients that help your body overcome the problems associated with excessive fat buildup. Trimbolic® supplies nutrients to help control binging and encourage your body to burn stored fat. A snack eaten between meals, Trimbolic® keeps you sustained until your next meal. Prevented from snacking, your body is forced to look to current stores of fat to use as fuel, thus igniting your body's natural furnace, your metabolism. Specific extracts help reduce the appearance of cellulite by enhancing the connective tissue structure and improving blood flow. Trimbolic® also slows down the body's absorption of sugar, preventing insulin excretion, again promoting fat loss. Trimbolic® is only available in my Transformation Weight Loss Program.

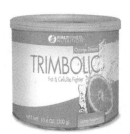

WEIGHT LOSS PROGRAM OVERVIEWS

Suddenly Slim — **Boost Weight Loss Program**, contains the combination of Reneú® and XanoLean™ Supreme. This program is ideal for individuals who need a quick jumpstart for their metabolism. Maybe you've been lax on your eating habits over the past few years, and as such, you've gained a few unwanted pounds. Reneú® will cleanse and detoxify your body, and XanoLean™ Supreme will help curb your appetite and support the fat burning process to get you results fast. Included in each of my programs is the nutritional menu guide, so you can learn how to make the right food choices to lose weight and feel great.

Suddenly Slim — **Accelerate Weight Loss Program**, contains the combination of Reneú®, XanoLean™ Supreme, and one canister of the perfect meal replacement protein shake, Body FX®. Replacing 14 meals, you don't have to worry about how you will get the essential protein and nutrients into your diet, because Body FX® is an immediate fix for fast food.

Suddenly Slim—Transformation Weight Loss Program is the all-in-one program. Incorporating my entire fleet of exclusive, doctor-recommended weight loss products, Reneú®, XanoLean™ Supreme, a canister of each flavor of Body FX®, replacing 28 meals, along with Trimbolic® you will lose the weight without counting calories, buying any fancy gym equipment, or starving yourself. A synergistic weight loss program, you can pick up the ultimate in *Suddenly Slim* Transformations.

30-Day Money-Back Guarantee: I am so proud of my product formulations and confident of the results you will achieve with the *Suddenly Slim* Weight Loss Program that if you aren't completely satisfied with the program, we offer a 30-day, no questions asked, money-back guarantee. If you are surprised we would put such a thing in writing, don't be. We have less than 1% of products returned!

SUPPLEMENT DIRECTIONS:

XanoLean™ Supreme: Take 1 caplet 3 times daily, approximately 45 minutes before meals, with a glass of water. For maximum weight loss results, do not skip 3rd caplet.

Reneú®: Take 1 to 2 capsules twice daily, before breakfast and at bedtime, with a glass of water. Start with 1 capsule and increase to 2 capsules as comfortable. Goal is 2 to 4 bowel movements per day.

Body FX®: Mix 2 level scoops (44 grams) of Body FX® into 8 oz. water, add ice, and blend well. For maximum weight loss results, use 2 shakes per day as a substitute for proteins.

Trimbolic®: Shake or briskly stir 1 level scoop Trimbolic® into 10 oz. chilled water. Drink immediately. Use mid-morning and mid-afternoon.

Included with each of my *Suddenly Slim* Weight Loss Programs is the *Suddenly Slim* Program and Menu Guide, which I have specifically designed to tell you exactly when to take which products. The Menu Guide is an incredibly simple-to-follow nutritional program. Yes, you will be eating real food. No counting calories, no weighing your food, and best of all, no starving. You will fuel your body with all of the high quality foods I've been teaching you about in this book at the right times of the day. My doctor-recommended supplements, paired with a nutritionally sound eating program, will enhance your weight loss results like never before.

Days 1 and 2: The first two days of the *Suddenly Slim* Weight Loss Program, sets your body up for accelerated weight loss. This is accomplished by focusing on the cleansing and detoxification process. This means adding in as few unknowns as possible. By incorporating 3 Body FX® meal replacement protein shakes a day (in addition to salads, unlimited thermic veggies, and snacks) instead of meats or other proteins, your body is able to access nutrients quickly and begin to absorb the protein, vitamins, and minerals from the Body FX® meal replacement protein shakes, which contain up to 50% of your recommended daily intake per serving. Your deficiency will be addressed directly with Body FX®, and you will be well on your way to a slimmer, healthier you in just 2 days on *Suddenly Slim*.

Days 3 through 10: These days allow for the incorporation of your preferred proteins for lunch and dinner. However, I have always recommended the use of 2 Body FX® meal replacement protein shakes a day to accelerate your weight loss results.

Days 11 through 30: You will notice on Day 11, we start to incorporate high-quality bread and grains back into your diet. While this is not a low carbohydrate diet by any stretch of the imagination, it is important to get your body working as efficiently as possible, as quickly as possible. Eliminating foods, even those that are healthy that hinder its overall efficiency, such as dairy, breads and grains, is the reasoning behind the first ten days of the 30-day program. Dairy and grains require extra facilities in the digestive process, while proteins and vegetables do not. Furthermore, for some, dairy and grains can cause digestive discomfort and/or bloating. Preventing the uninhibited flow of nutrients, my program allows your body to get back to the basic building blocks and lock in all of the required nutrients your body has been missing.

Drink Lots of Water: While we had an entire chapter on the importance of water, I would be amiss if I didn't reiterate the importance of water within our program. Take your starting weight, cut that number in half and add 8 to this number. This is how much water, in ounces, you should be drinking daily. If you need to lose more than 25 pounds, add an additional 8 ounces of water to your daily intake for every 25 pounds that you want to lose.

In the next chapter you will learn how to transition from getting *Suddenly Slim*, to staying *Suddenly Slim*. But first, I want to thank you for making it this far. You should be immensely proud of yourself. Taking the next step isn't always easy, but the thing about the next step is that it allows you to look back on how far you've come, which is always an amazing feeling. Progress isn't measured by perfection, but in a series of small steps. This, for you, is one of those steps. Welcome to *Suddenly Slim*.

CHAPTER 8: TAKEAWAYS

1. The cornerstone of a healthy body relies on detoxification and cleansing. Cleansing the body of toxins and impurities is paramount in helping you absorb essential nutrients.

2. Enjoy Body FX® 1-3 times daily. The perfect meal, Body FX® will ensure your macronutrient needs are met without you having to count a single calorie.

3. Supplement your diet with one of the most powerful fat burners on the market. XanoLean™ Supreme should be taken 3x daily, 45 minutes before meals, for maximum results.

4. Trimbolic®, the ultimate cellulite fighter, works best in between meals to help keep you satisfied.

5. My Menu Guide provides real-world options for you to lose weight and not be hungry.

6. With the unlimited consumption of thermic veggies, not only will you have plentiful food, unlike other programs, you will learn how to cook and eat nutritious foods.

CHAPTER 9

STAY
SUDDENLY SLIM®

After completing your first 30 days on a *Suddenly Slim* Weight Loss Program, there are generally 2 types of people: those who still have more weight to lose and others who have achieved their weight loss goals.

WANT TO LOSE MORE WEIGHT?

For those of you who still need to lose more weight, I recommend you stay on your *Suddenly Slim* 30-Day Program until you reach your desired weight loss results. However, start your next 30-Day Program, with Day 11 and continue for the rest of your weight-loss journey.

HAVE YOU HIT A WEIGHT-LOSS PLATEAU?

I categorize a weight-loss plateau as more than 3 days where you haven't lost weight or inches. If you have hit a weight loss plateau, don't worry. This happens. Your body is incredibly smart at adapting, and you just need a quick reset. If this occurs to you, start the Program over at Day 1. Continue to weigh according to the same schedule as your first Program: days 1, 4, 7, 11, 18, 25, and 30.

MAINTAIN YOUR WEIGHT LOSS

To maintain your weight loss, it is important to continue to swap at least one meal a day with Body FX®, which is the Holy Grail of balanced nutrition. Your new body needs to continue to receive essential nutrients to stay healthy, and Body FX® is the solution.

I also encourage you to continue use of Reneú®. Your interaction with toxins and chemicals hasn't decreased, you've just cleaned out the current backlog. To keep the weight off, and continue to reap the benefits of a healthy inner body and colon, you need to supplement Reneú® accordingly. I suggest one to two capsules daily.

And for those predisposed to crave foods and snacks, XanoLean Supreme™ is a safe fat burner to quell cravings, and I advocate for a *use as needed* protocol. Using as needed will allow you more control on days you need it, like Thanksgiving, Christmas, New Year's, and other popular food-enriched holidays.

THE POWER OF VEGETABLES

It is important to eat a variety of fruits and vegetables every day. Some thermic veggies lower your risk of heart disease, while others lower your risk of cancers. We need to fuel our body with as many phytochemicals as possible, natural compounds found in produce that help slow the aging process, which is an outcome we can all jump aboard. The wider the variety of fruits and vegetables you consume, the better balanced your macronutrient and micronutrient portfolio will be. Plus, eating unlimited vegetables during the day will help to maintain your weight and keep you full. Stick to the thermic vegetables on the *Suddenly*

> **IT IS IMPORTANT TO EAT A VARIETY OF FRUITS AND VEGETABLES EVERY DAY.**

POSITIVE SELF-TALK

Your mindset is the most powerful physiological weight-loss tool and arguably one of the most important tools overall. Self-talk is the endless stream of unspoken thoughts that run through our minds. Positive or negative, these thoughts can come from logic and reason, while others stem from a poisoned view of yourself, or the world around you. This is comparable to having a glass half-full or glass half-empty mentality. It is important to be rational and realistic, but being overwhelmingly negative benefits no one, yourself included. Tremendous health benefits are attributed to positive thinking: increased life span, reduced rates of depression, increased coping skills, and a reduced risk for cardiovascular disease. In addition to those health benefits, manifesting positive vibes and creating what could be a new outlook on your life, positive self-talk has shown to reduce stress. Stress reduction, no matter how it's done, is **huge** for your overall health and weight loss!

Well, how do I know what negative self-talk is? I think from time to time, we all experience some degree of negative self-talk, but it's important to identify negative self-talk and develop a plan of attack for when it inevitably pops into your head. By magnifying the negative aspects of a situation, you squash anything good resulting from it. If you are open to positivity, you can find the light in almost every situation. My life could have been dramatically different if I had chosen to let how unfair my life began control my thoughts. I am so thankful polio's devastating effects stopped at the physical level and didn't plunge me into a pool of darkness. If you open your mind and let some light in, the possibilities are truly endless.

DE-STRESS YOUR LIFE

Stress takes a major toll on your health. We each face a mounting list of demands from both our personal and professional life on a daily basis. Minor hassles may seem insignificant, but with each new addition, your body begins to prep for an assault or threat to its overall well-being. In anticipation, your body resorts to releasing a well-known hormone, cortisol. Signaled for release by the hypothalamus in your brain, your adrenal glands release a dose of cortisol, usually accompanied by another well-known hormone, adrenaline, the fight-or-flight hormone.

Adrenaline is released to increase your focus and boost energy supplies during times that you should be in immediate danger. That is just how powerful stress can be. It literally makes your body believe you are being threatened! While adrenaline is being released, it's joined by cortisol, which increases the amount of glucose that flows in your blood. However, it doesn't stop there. Cortisol down regulates functions that your body doesn't need in a fight-or-flight type of situation, such as the reproductive system, the growth processes and—you guessed it —the digestive system. So you have all of this sugar in your blood, and your body has no way to make use of it. Unlike adrenaline, which is only active for short bursts, cortisol has put forth a chain of events that isn't as easy to simply turn off. It's paramount you learn how to deal with essential stresses of your life and find a way to relieve your stress like yoga or another form of working out, enjoying a long walk around the neighborhood, listening to music, reading a book—anything that allows you to unwind.

While some stress is unavoidable, most is unnecessary. Try and rid unneeded stress from your life. This doesn't mean you have to cut friends and family out of your life, but maybe it means you need to sit down and have a heart-to-heart with them. Invite them into your new world and kindly explain to them how important it is you surround yourself with positivity. As a direct result of the conversation, they will just pay closer attention to what they project and their desire to better themselves in light of your goals.

VERBALIZE YOUR GOALS

In order to continue your healthy lifestyle, it's important you become accountable, either by finding a friend who can help you stay on track during a particularly rough time or just talking with your friends and family about your goals. Verbalization of our goals is one of the most important steps in success for all things in life. It allows those around us to really offer their support. People are not mind readers, nor can we rely on subtle messages and dropping hints. Just starting a weight loss program doesn't signal to those around you that you are serious about getting healthy. And just as with most things in life, a support system is crucial for success. There will be times when you had a rough day, and your old habits attempt a comeback. If they do, wouldn't it be nice to have your significant other remind you that ice cream will not help you reach your goals? Also, it is proven you will have much better weight loss results if you start your weight-loss journey with a friend. Whom would you like to share this life-changing opportunity with?

HOLD YOURSELF ACCOUNTABLE

In addition to personal support, you need to be able to rely on yourself. Knowing why you want to get healthy is sometimes all you need to get the job done, but acknowledging you have the

THINK BACK TO YOUR "WHY," AND OFTEN.

power to lose the weight is incredibly motivating. It all begins with your "Why." Think back to your "Why," and often. I urge you to strongly consider starting a motivational board. Fill it with goals from all areas of your life: from your family, to your job, to your health. Save photos, make plans, and map out your life's successes before they happen. That which you manifest becomes true.

WEIGHING IN

Make sure you measure, weigh, and take progress photos often. I recommend weighing on days 1, 4, 7, 11, 18, 25, and 30 while on the *Suddenly Slim* Program. Remember inch loss is better than actual weight loss. Your weight loss might not always come from your waist; sometimes we lose weight in our face or other areas we can't really measure through traditional methods. Photos become especially important when you add working out into your weight loss regimen. When you are new to a healthy lifestyle that includes exercise, like lifting weights or running, you almost always enjoy the perks of what is called body recomposition. A technical term for reshaping your body, this is what happens when your body converts fat into muscle. A major bonus, muscle is much more compact than fat, meaning the scale might not move, but when you measure yourself, and look at photos you can see inch loss. The bottom line is, while a great tool, don't solely rely on the scale as confirmation you are losing fat. There are a number of reasons

I RECOMMEND WEIGHING ON DAYS 1, 4, 7, 11, 18, 25, AND 30 WHILE ON THE *SUDDENLY SLIM* PROGRAM.

why your scale weight would be up but you have lost fat. Instead, rely on your tape measure, your eyes, and your clothing. Nothing says fat loss quite like buttoning up on a pair of jeans that you couldn't last month. Once you have lost the weight, it is important to continue to weigh yourself frequently enough to make sure you are on track, but daily weighing is not good for you. It can cause you to become overly paranoid or concerned with a number, something I do not advocate.

EXERCISE

Try to exercise 3 to 4 times a week for at least 30 minutes. Exercising increases your metabolism, builds lean muscle tissue, and provides an overall feeling of well-being. Even a 30-minute brisk walk is beneficial. Gaining just one extra pound of muscle can allow you to burn an extra 30–50 calories every single day! Consider joining a local gym. Most gyms offer group classes from yoga, to full body, or even a beginner's guide to weight lifting.

TRY TO EXERCISE 3 TO 4 TIMES A WEEK FOR AT LEAST 30-MINUTES.

I strongly encourage this form of interaction, especially if you're a newcomer to the fitness world. These group classes allow you to learn basics, such as form and execution, and encourage friendships with people whose interests align with yours. If you are shy, there are also numerous at home workouts you can do, both through YouTube or for purchase.

CHAPTER 9: TAKEAWAYS

1. Incorporate positive self-talk. Believe in yourself and the possibilities are limitless.

2. Develop a strong support system by vocalizing your goals to your friends, family, and the other people in your life. Without their help, you will find yourself in an uphill battle.

3. Repeat the *Suddenly Slim* Weight Loss Program of your choice as often as desired. It is completely safe and backed by doctors. Don't let life get in the way of a healthy, slim you.

4. Rid yourself of stress and, if possible, stressful people.

5. Adhere to the *Suddenly Slim* Program "weigh-in" days. Including measurements and photos, weighing in allows you to see your progress. Nothing sparks motivation quite like seeing results.

6. Begin to research ways you can add working out and exercise into your weekly routine.

WEIGHT LOSS SUCCESS TIPS

COOK AT HOME

Frequently cooking at home will ensure you have as much control as possible over what you put in your body. Be sure to bring the menu guide with you to the grocery store. Key to success #1: if it's not on the Menu Guide, do not buy it!

Most cooking sprays note they have 0 calories, but how can this be when they are oil based? In the US, if a product has less than 5 grams of fat per serving, the total fat content can be rounded to the nearest .5g. So in the case of cooking sprays, if you go over the suggested serving size, which is a quick spritz, or 1/3 of a second, you will in fact be getting extra calories. In fact, most of us spray at least 3 to 6 times too long!

Drain your meat before adding it to your plate. In doing so, you could eliminate your intake of an extra 4 grams of fat per 3-ounce serving! This can be accomplished by either rinsing your meat once it is transferred into the colander, or just allowing it to sit in the colander for a few extra minutes.

Stick to baking, roasting, and stir-frying as preparation methods.

Before you start cooking, wash your produce! Pesticides from fruit and vegetables have been proven to slow down the metabolism. It's important you scrub fresh produce for at least 30 seconds to remove any residue before eating. As noted in previous chapters, buying locally grown and organic can dramatically reduce the amount of pesticides on foods, especially those that have an edible peel.

On the subject of vegetables, a recent study by Penn State confirmed that people who frequently incorporated vegetables into their main dish consumed 350 fewer calories a day than those who only had a veggie as a side.

Devote a couple of hours one day a week to prep your meals for the upcoming week. Ensuring you have portioned out proteins, salads, and vegetables at the ready will allow you to stick to your plan. I am sure you are familiar with the *hangry* feeling and reaching for the first thing you can find. If you are really strapped for time, you can even put together weeks' worth of food in bulk, freezing each individual meal until you need it.

For dinners, make use of a slow cooker. Take one of those aforementioned preprepped meals from the freezer, put it in the old slow cooker before you leave for work, cook on low for 8 hours, and when you get home, you have a freshly prepared meal waiting for you! Tremendous meal options with the slow cooker are available with little to no effort! Just one can of broth, loads of veggies, and a breast of chicken seasoned right can be a delicious meal, with a minimal amount of prep time.

EATING OUT TIPS

Once you've lost the weight, keeping it off and eating out is possible. I have several tricks that once you master will allow you to join friends and family at plenty of restaurants.

If the ingredients from the menu guide are on a dish from the restaurant, chances are they can make special accommodations for you. Call ahead to find out if they can and keep track of restaurants who are friendly to your weight maintenance goals for future reference, avoiding buffets and restaurants offering all-you-can-eat options.

Before you leave for a dinner, always have a scoop of Body FX®
before you go. Far too often we wait until we are far too hungry
before we eat. Having just one scoop, half a serving of Body
FX®, will ensure your blood sugar stays level and that you don't
overeat.

Ask the server to NOT bring bread to the table. It is far easier to
ask them to skip the bread than it is to resist its temptation.

Look at the salad options first. They often include a nice selection
of on Menu Guide options. But before ordering, confirm with
your server all of the ingredients the salad contains. Sometimes
restaurants add in small amounts of bacon, cheese, or other
ingredients that are not listed in the menu.

Always ask for dressings/sauces on the side. Use your fork to
dip in the ramekin of dressing/sauce, and then pick up a bite
with your fork. With this method, you will use far less and still get
ample flavor.

Request a to-go box to accompany your meal. Once your meal
arrives, immediately split it up into halves and pack one half to
go.

Try to eat slowly. Chewing each bite 40 times, as compared to the
average of 15, lowers ghrelin levels. In addition, the further you
break down food before it enters your digestive track, the more
nutrients you will receive. Slowing down also allows your stomach
to catch up to your mouth. It's estimated that it takes about 20
minutes for your brain to register your stomach is full. If we stop
eating when we feel we are full, we will actually be overfull 20
minutes later.

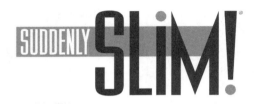

REAL **PEOPLE!** REAL **RESULTS!**

And now, if you haven't already skipped ahead, here is a compilation of *Suddenly Slim* Weight Loss Program success stories. These individuals poured their hearts and souls into their transformations, and I couldn't be prouder. I hope to see you in one of these in the very near future. To order your *Suddenly Slim* Weight Loss Program, contact your FirstFitness Nutrition Independent Distributor at GetSuddenlySlim.com.

NAME: **NUMBER:**

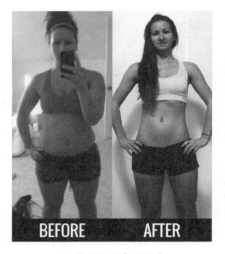

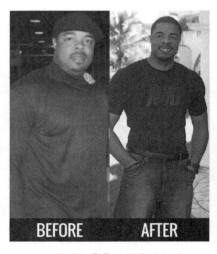

I LOST **50 LBS**
AND **42 INCHES!**
– ASHLEY R.

I LOST **98 LBS** AND
60 INCHES IN **8 MONTHS!**
– TORRANCE N.

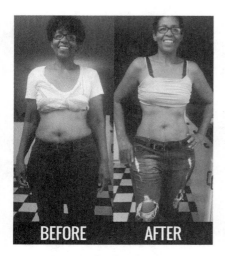

BEFORE   AFTER

I LOST **10.2 LBS** AND
21 INCHES IN **30 DAYS!**
— WANDA L.

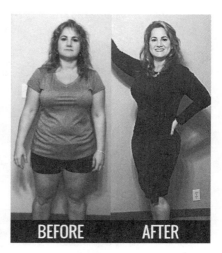

BEFORE   AFTER

I LOST **13.5** AND
18.25 INCHES IN **30 DAYS!**
— FELISA C.

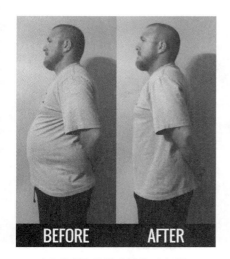

BEFORE   AFTER

I LOST **15 LBS** AND
11.25 INCHES IN **30 DAYS!**
— JOHN C.

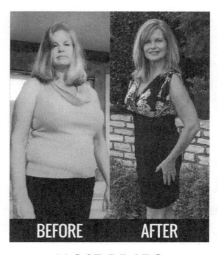

BEFORE   AFTER

I LOST **15 LBS**
AND **21 INCHES!**
— JANET E.

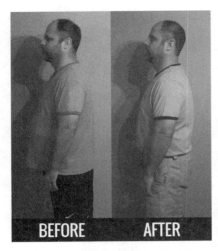

I LOST **20.4 LBS** AND
14.5 INCHES IN **30 DAYS!**
– DARRELL D.

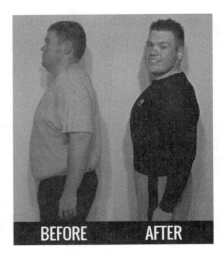

I LOST **21 LBS** AND
15 INCHES IN **30 DAYS!**
– LANE E.

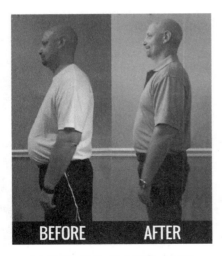

I LOST **21.5 LBS** AND
12 INCHES IN **30 DAYS!**
– FRANKIE T.

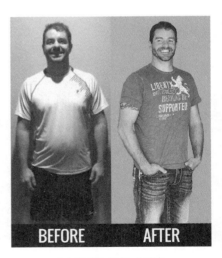

I LOST **22 LBS**
AND **11 INCHES!**
– LLOYD H.

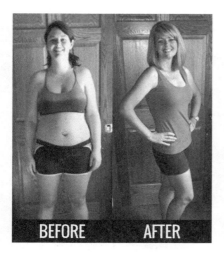

I LOST **22 LBS**
AND **19 INCHES!**
– RACHEL J.

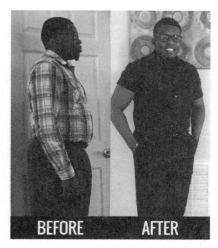

I LOST **23.4 LBS** AND
14 INCHES IN **30 DAYS!**
– ALTON S.

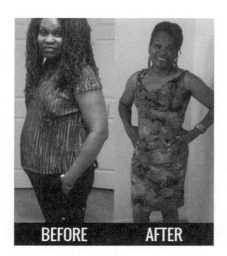

I LOST **25 LBS**
AND **30 INCHES!**
– MARILYN B.

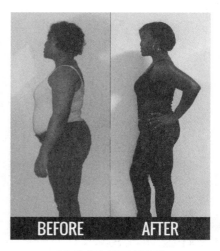

I LOST **27 LBS**
AND **39 INCHES!**
– DEWANDA R.

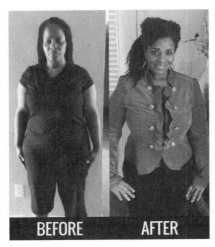

I LOST **32 LBS** AND **21 INCHES** IN **30 DAYS!**
– TUNDA W.

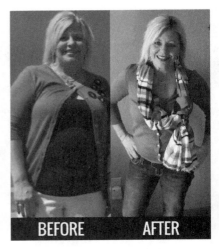

I LOST **48 LBS** AND **47 INCHES!**
– TRACEY C.

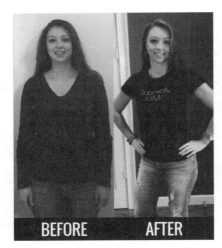

I LOST **50 LBS** AND **46 INCHES!**
– MELINDA A.

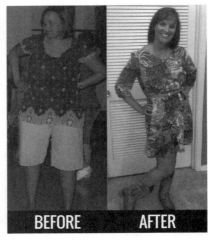

I LOST **60 LBS** AND **22 LBS** IN **30 DAYS!**
– JENNIFER E.

These results are not typical. Weight loss varies with each individual depending upon a variety of factors.
All testimonies may or may not be representative of the actual weight you can lose with FirstFitness Nutrition products.

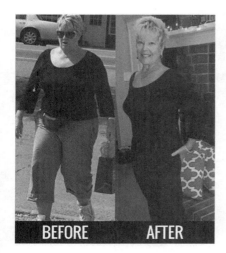

BEFORE   **AFTER**

I LOST **65 LBS**
AND **47 INCHES!**
– DONNA C.

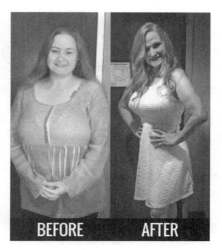

BEFORE   **AFTER**

I LOST
70 LBS!
– LAJUANA G.

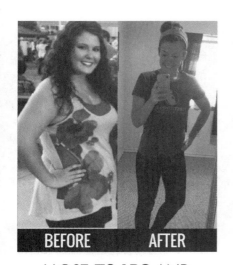

BEFORE   **AFTER**

I LOST **70 LBS** AND
31 LBS IN **30 DAYS!**
– JORDAN B.

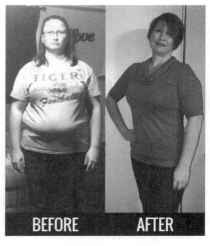

BEFORE   **AFTER**

I LOST **70 LBS** AND
50 INCHES IN **5 MONTHS!**
– KRISTY C.

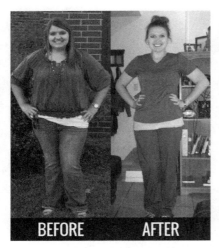

I LOST **72 LBS**
AND **47 INCHES!**
– AMBER B.

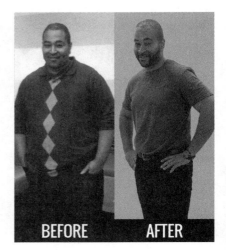

I LOST
100 LBS!
– DAVID G.

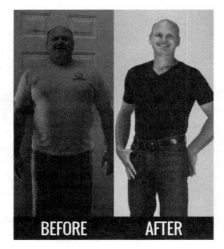

I LOST
100 LBS!
– JEFF P.

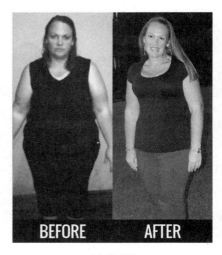

I LOST
100 LBS!
– DEHLIA C.

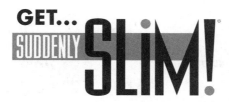

RECIPE COLLECTION

For most people, the key to successfully losing weight and keeping it off is developing a new mindset and a healthy attitude and approach toward food. We need to replace the existing mindset of food as needed for socialization, boredom, or a reward. Food is, and should be viewed as, a fuel resource. If we fill our bodies with the right fuel, we will get the right energy and the ability to stay healthy and lean in exchange.

Bad habits are hard to break, but when you know how to properly prepare healthy foods, you will be amazed at not only how easy it is to eat clean, but how delicious, too.

Here is just one of the many places our #GetSuddenlySlim community steps in and supports you in your weight loss journey. Our amazing scientists, medical professionals, and nutritionists have put together Suddenly Slim Program friendly recipe after delicious recipe, proven to help you stay on track and achieve your goals. With more than 70 recipes, from amazing protein meal replacements shakes to nutritious meals and filling snacks, you can mix up your meals as much or as little as you like!

I hope you enjoy these recipes as much as I do!

Lee Causey

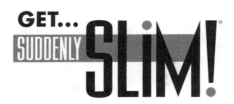

RECIPE COLLECTION

SHAKES:
Breakfast Shakes
Lunch & Dinner Shakes

VEGETABLES

DRESSINGS

LUNCH & DINNER:
Beef
Chicken
Fish
Soup
Turkey
Vegetarian

BREADS & GRAINS
Enjoy on/after Day 11...

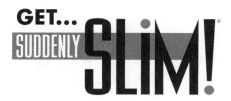

SHAKE RECIPES

BREAKFAST SHAKES | ENJOY DAYS 1 – 30

Apple Pie

Berry Good

Blueberry Dream

Chocolate Covered Strawberries

Double Berry

Raspberry Truffle

Rise & Shine

Strawberry Banana

Strawberry Supreme

Triple Berry

Very Blueberry

Wild About Berries

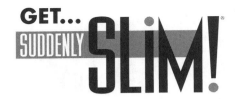

BREAKFAST SHAKES

APPLE PIE

Ingredients
- 2 scoops Body FX® Tropical Crème
- 1/2 cup chopped apple
- 8-10 oz. water
- dash cinnamon
- dash nutmeg
- ice, optional

Directions
Mix all ingredients together and blend.

BERRY GOOD

Ingredients
- 2 scoops Body FX® Tropical Crème
- 1/3 cup strawberries
- 8-10 oz. water
- 1/3 cup blueberries
- 1/3 cup blackberries
- ice, optional

Directions
Mix all ingredients together and blend.

BLUEBERRY DREAM

Ingredients
- 2 scoops Body FX® Tropical Crème
- 1 cup blueberries
- ice, optional
- 8-10 oz. water

Directions
Mix all ingredients together and blend.

CHOCOLATE COVERED STRAWBERRIES

Ingredients
- 2 scoops Body FX® Chocolate Paradise
- 1 cup strawberries
- 8-10 oz. water
- ice, optional

Directions
Mix all ingredients together and blend.

DOUBLE BERRY

Ingredients
- 2 scoops Body FX® Tropical Crème
- 1/2-cup strawberries
- 8-10 oz. water
- 1/2 cup blueberries
- ice, optional

Directions
Mix all ingredients together and blend.

RASPBERRY TRUFFLE

Ingredients
- 2 scoops Body FX® Tropical Crème
- 2 tsp. raspberry extract
- 8-10 oz. water
- 1 cup raspberries
- ice, optional

Directions
Mix all ingredients together and blend.

RISE & SHINE

Ingredients
- 2 scoops Body FX® Tropical Crème
- 1 selection of fresh or frozen fruit from menu guide
- 8-10 oz. water
- ice, optional

Directions
Mix all ingredients together and blend.

STRAWBERRY BANANA

Ingredients
- 2 scoops Body FX® Tropical Crème
- 1 tbsp. sugar-free banana pudding mix
- ice, optional
- 1 cup strawberries
- 8-10 oz. water

Directions
Mix all ingredients together and blend.

STRAWBERRY SUPREME

Ingredients
- 2 scoops Body FX® Tropical Crème
- 1 cup strawberries
- 8-10 oz. water
- ice, optional

Directions
Mix all ingredients together and blend.

TRIPLE BERRY

Ingredients
- 2 scoops Body FX® Tropical Crème
- 3 medium strawberries
- 8-10 oz. water
- 1/4 cup blackberries
- 1/4 cup raspberries
- ice, optional

Directions
Mix all ingredients together and blend.

WILD ABOUT BERRIES

Ingredients
- 2 scoops Body FX® Tropical Crème
- 4 strawberries
- 8-10 oz. water
- 6-8 raspberries
- 15 blueberries
- ice, optional

Directions
Mix all ingredients together and blend.

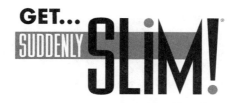

SHAKE RECIPES

LUNCH/DINNER SHAKES | ENJOY DAYS 1-30

Amaretto Joy
Bahama Breeze
Chocolate Frappuccino
Cinnamon Roll
Go Bananas
Green Machine
Hot Cappuccino
Lemon Cooler
Orange Dreamsicle Delight
Peanut Butter Banana*
Peanut Butter Brittle*
Peanut Butter Chocolate*
Piña Colada
Pumpkin Pie
Pumpkin Spice Protein Latte
The Hulk
Tropical Breeze

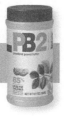

*These recipes contain PB2 (powdered peanut butter) which can be purchased at Wal-Mart, Amazon, or any health food store.

101

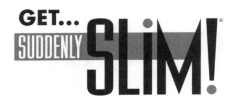

LUNCH & DINNER SHAKES

AMARETTO JOY

Ingredients
- 2 scoops Body FX® Tropical Crème
- 8-10 oz. water
- 1 tsp. of almond extract
- ice, optional

Directions
Mix all ingredients together and blend.

BAHAMA BREEZE

Ingredients
- 2 scoops Body FX® Tropical Crème
- 1 tbsp. sugar-free gelatin orange mix
- 8-10 oz. water
- 1 tsp. rum extract
- 1 tsp. coconut extract
- ice, optional

Directions
Mix all ingredients together and blend.

CHOCOLATE FRAPPUCCINO

Ingredients
- 2 scoops Body FX® Chocolate Paradise
- 8-10 oz. cold coffee
- ice, optional

Directions
Mix all ingredients together and blend.

CINNAMON ROLL

Ingredients
- 2 scoops Body FX® Tropical Crème
- dash cinnamon
- 8-10 oz. water
- 1/2 cup chopped apple
- dash nutmeg
- ice, optional

Directions
Mix all ingredients together and blend.

GO BANANAS

Ingredients
- 2 scoops Body FX® Tropical Crème
- 1 tbsp. sugar-free banana pudding mix
- 8-10 oz. water
- ice, optional

Directions
Mix all ingredients together and blend.

GREEN MACHINE

Ingredients
- 2 scoops Body FX® Tropical Crème
- 8-10 oz. water
- handful of spinach
- ice, optional

Directions
Mix all ingredients together and blend.

HOT CHOCOLATE CAPPUCCINO

Ingredients
- 2 scoops Body FX® Chocolate Paradise
- 1 cup coffee
- 8-10 oz. of boiling water

Directions
Mix all ingredients together and blend.

LEMON COOLER

Ingredients
- 2 scoops Body FX® Tropical Crème
- 8-10 oz. water
- 2 tsp. lemon juice
- ice, optional

Directions
Mix all ingredients together and blend.

ORANGE DREAMSICLE DELIGHT

Ingredients
- 2 scoops Body FX® Tropical Crème
- 1 tsp. sugar-free orange gelatin mix
- 8-10 oz. water
- ice, optional

Directions
Mix all ingredients together and blend.

PEANUT BUTTER BANANA

Ingredients
- 2 scoops Body FX® Chocolate Paradise
- 1 tbsp. PB2 (powdered peanut butter)
- 1 tbsp. sugar-free banana pudding mix
- 8-10 oz. water
- ice, optional

Directions
Mix all ingredients together and blend.

PEANUT BUTTER BRITTLE

Ingredients
- 2 scoops Body FX® Tropical Crème
- 1 tbsp. PB2 (powdered peanut butter)
- 1 tbsp. sugar-free butterscotch pudding mix
- 8-10 oz. water
- ice, optional

Directions
Mix all ingredients together and blend.

PEANUT BUTTER CHOCOLATE

Ingredients
- 2 scoops Body FX® Chocolate Paradise
- 1 tbsp. PB2 (powdered peanut butter)
- 8-10 oz. water
- ice, optional

Directions
Mix all ingredients together and blend.

PIÑA COLADA

Ingredients
- 2 scoops Body FX® Tropical Crème
- 1/2 tsp. coconut extract
- 1 tsp. pineapple extract
- 8-10 oz. of water

Directions
Mix all ingredients together and blend.

PUMPKIN PIE

Ingredients
- 2 scoops Body FX® Tropical Crème
- 2 tbsp. canned pumpkin, no sugar added
- pumpkin spice, to taste
- cinnamon, to taste
- 8-10 oz. water
- ice, optional

Directions
Mix all ingredients together and blend.

PUMPKIN SPICE PROTEIN LATTE

Ingredients
- 1 scoop Body FX® Tropical Crème
- 1/4 cup canned pumpkin, no sugar added
- 1/8 tsp. pumpkin spice
- 1/2 cup skim milk
- 1/8 tsp. cinnamon
- 6-8 oz. coffee

Directions
Mix all ingredients together and blend.

THE HULK

Ingredients
- 2 scoops Body FX® Tropical Crème
- 1/2 tbsp. sugar-free pistachio pudding mix
- handful of spinach
- 8-10 oz. water
- ice, optional

Directions
Mix all ingredients together and blend.

TROPICAL BREEZE

Ingredients
- 2 scoops Body FX® Tropical Crème
- 1 tsp. sugar-free strawberry gelatin mix
- 1 tsp. sugar-free lime gelatin mix
- 1 tsp. sugar-free orange gelatin mix
- 8-10 oz. water
- ice, optional

Directions
Mix all ingredients together and blend.

VANILLA FRAPPUCCINO

Ingredients
- 2 scoops Body FX® Tropical Crème
- 8-10 oz. cold coffee
- ice, optional

Directions
Mix all ingredients together and blend.

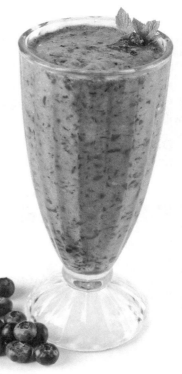

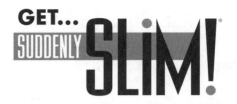

VEGETABLE RECIPES

ENJOY DAYS 1-30

Butternut Squash Fries

Cauliflower Rice

Cauliflower Mashed Potatoes

Garlic Roasted Brussels Sprouts

Green Beans with Creamy Garlic Dressing

Italian Tomato Basil Zucchini Pasta

Spicy Garlic Broccoli

Squash Chips

Stir Fried Green Beans

Zesty Cucumbers

BUTTERNUT SQUASH FRIES | 1 SERVING

Ingredients
- 1/2 butternut squash, peeled, seeded, and cut into steak fry sized pieces
- 2 tbsp. extra-virgin olive oil
- Any mix of spices including but not limited to: chili powder, paprika, cayenne pepper, sea salt, and pepper

Directions
1. Preheat oven to 425°F.
2. In a big bowl or Ziploc bag, add the fries and olive oil, then toss to coat.
3. Add seasonings, toss to coat, again.
4. Line a cookie sheet with parchment paper and put fries on sheet in a single layer.
5. Bake for 20 minutes, flip fries & bake for another 15-20 minutes.
6. Broil on each side for 1-2 minutes.

Suddenly Slim **Recipe Box**

CAULIFLOWER RICE | 1 SERVING

Ingredients
- 1 head cauliflower, any size
- 1 tbsp. extra-virgin olive oil or butter, optional
- sea salt and pepper

Directions
1. Cut cauliflower into large pieces.
2. Transfer cauliflower to food processor or blender.
3. Pulse or blend until cauliflower is broken down into tiny pieces.
4. Warm olive oil or butter in large skillet over medium heat.
5. Stir in cauliflower and sprinkle with seasoning.
6. Cover and cook for 5 to 8 minutes, or until desired texture.

Adapted from **The Kitchn**

CAULIFLOWER MASHED POTATOES | 6 - 8 SERVINGS

Ingredients

- 1 large head of cauliflower
- 2 tbsp. of butter
- 5 large cloves of garlic, minched
- 1/4 tsp. nutmeg
- sea salt and pepper to taste

Directions

1. Bring a large stock pot to boil over high heat.
2. Thoroughly wash and cut cauliflower into small pieces.
3. Cook cauliflower in water for 6 minutes or until very well done.
4. Drain and pat dry before the cauliflower cools.
5. In a food processor, or with blender in batches, puree the hot cauliflower with remaining ingredients until smooth.

Suddenly Slim **Recipe Box**

GARLIC ROASTED BRUSSELS SPROUTS | 2 SERVINGS

Ingredients

- 1 pound Brussels sprouts
- 4 tbsp. extra-virgin olive oil
- 2 tsp. lemon juice
- 1 garlic cloves, minced
- 1/2 tsp. cayenne pepper
- sea salt, to taste

Directions

1. Preheat oven to 400°F.
2. Bring large pot of lightly salted water to a boil. Add Brussels sprouts and cook for two minutes. Drain well and place the sprouts in a large bowl.
3. Add the minced garlic, cayenne pepper, and olive oil and gently toss to coat. Transfer the sprouts to a baking pan and sprinkle with sea salt. Bake for 15-20 minutes, shaking pan occasionally, until sprouts are quite brown and crisp on the outside and tender on the inside.
4. Adjust the taste with more sea salt if necessary. Drizzle with lemon juice, toss to combine and serve.

Submitted by **Reneé Eads**

GREEN BEANS WITH CREAMY GARLIC DRESSING
2 - 4 SERVINGS

Ingredients
- 1 lb. green beans, trimmed and cut diagonally into 1-inch pieces
- 1 small clove garlic, minced, or 1/2 tsp. garlic powder
- 1/2 tsp. sea salt
- 1/2 cup nonfat plain yogurt
- 1 tbsp. extra-virgin olive oil
- 1 tbsp. chopped fresh parsley, (optional)
- freshly ground pepper, to taste

Directions
1. Place a medium bowl of ice water near the stove. Bring an inch of water to a boil in a large saucepan fitted with a steamer basket. Add green beans, cover, and cook until tender, 6 to 8 minutes. Transfer the beans to the ice water to cool. Remove from the ice water with a slotted spoon and let drain on a kitchen towel; blot dry with another towel.
2. If using fresh garlic, mash with salt using the back of a spoon until a paste forms. Whisk the garlic paste (or garlic powder and sea salt) with yogurt, oil, parsley (if using), and pepper in a large bowl. Add the green beans and toss to coat. Serve chilled.

Adapted from **Eatingwell.com**

ITALIAN TOMATO BASIL ZUCCHINI PASTA
2 SERVINGS

Ingredients
- 2 zucchinis
- 1/2 lemon
- 5 fresh basil leaves
- 2 tomatoes
- 1 tsp. extra-virgin olive oil
- sea salt, to taste

Directions
1. Use a vegetable peeler to make the fettuccine noodles.
2. Stop peeling when you get down to the seeds.
3. Dice the center portion of the zucchini and add it to the bowl along with the noodles.
4. Chop the tomatoes and add them to the bowl.
5. Slice the basil leaves as small as possible and add to the bowl.
6. Squeeze the 1/2 lemon. Add a little olive oil. Sprinkle with a little sea salt. Mix it up and serve.
7. The longer it sits, the softer the noodles become.

Suddenly Slim **Recipe Box**

SQUASH CHIPS | 1 - 2 SERVINGS

Ingredients
- Squash, sliced 1/4" thick
- extra-virgin olive oil cooking spray
- sea salt, to taste

Directions
1. Preheat oven to 350°F.
2. Spray squash slices on both sides with olive oil cooking spray.
3. Lightly sea salt and bake slices slowly until they are crisp and light brown.
4. Watch closely to avoid over baking.

Suddenly Slim **Recipe Box**

STIR FRIED GREEN BEANS | 2 - 4 SERVINGS

Ingredients
- 1/2 pound green beans
- 1 tbsp. garlic, minced
- 1 tsp. Bragg's Amino Acids (or light soy sauce)
- 1 tbsp. butter or coconut oil
- 1/2 tsp. sea salt

Directions
1. Heat frying pan or wok to medium high heat. Add coconut oil or butter and minced garlic.
2. When garlic begins to brown slightly, add green beans.
3. Add 1 tbsp. water, cover, and steam.
4. Wait about 5 minutes, or until beans are cooked through. Add sea salt and Bragg's or soy sauce to taste.

Submitted by **Coletta Hakenewerth**

ZESTY CUCUMBERS | 1 SERVING

Ingredients
- 1 cucumber
- 1 lime
- 1 tsp. chili powder

Directions
1. Squeeze lime juice over chopped cucumbers and sprinkle with chili powder.

Suddenly Slim **Recipe Box**

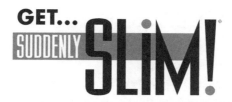

DRESSING RECIPES

ENJOY DAYS 1 - 30

Creamy Cilantro Avocado Dressing

Chipotle Ranch Dressing

Tomato-Paprika Salad Dressing

CREAMY CILANTRO AVOCADO DRESSING

Ingredients
- 1 cup loosely packed cilantro, stems removed & roughly chopped
- 1/2 avocado
- 1 tbsp. fresh lime juice (1/2 lime), more to taste
- 1-2 garlic cloves
- 1/4 cup extra-virgin olive oil
- 1 1/2 tsp. water
- 1/8 tsp. sea salt

Directions
1. Put all ingredients in food processor and puree about one minute with steel blade.

Submitted by **Wendy Miller**

CHIPOTLE RANCH DRESSING

Ingredients
- 2 cups light ranch dressing
- 1/2 cup chunky salsa
- 1/2 tsp. ground chipotle chili powder

Directions
1. Put salsa in food processor and puree about one minute with steel blade.
2. Add light ranch dressing and ground chipotle and process 30 seconds more, or until well combined.

Suddenly Slim **Recipe Box**

TOMATO-PAPRIKA SALAD DRESSING

Ingredients
- 3/4 pound plum or other ripe tomatoes
- 3 tbsp. red-wine vinegar
- 1 to 2 tsp. light-brown sugar substitute
- 1 small clove garlic, roughly chopped
- 1/2 tsp. mild paprika
- 1/4 cup extra-virgin olive oil
- sea salt and ground pepper, to taste

Directions
1. With a paring knife, cut a shallow x in the bottom of the tomatoes. Bring a medium saucepan of water to a boil. Add tomatoes and boil 30 seconds. Using a slotted spoon, transfer tomatoes to a bowl. When cool enough to handle, peel and discard their skin. Cut tomatoes into quarters lengthwise. Using your fingers, discard seeds. Transfer tomatoes to a blender.
2. Add vinegar, sugar, garlic, and paprika and puree until smooth. Remove the center cap, and with the motor running, add olive oil in a steady stream. Season with sea salt and pepper.

Suddenly Slim **Recipe Box**

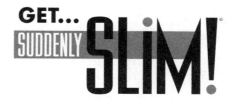

LUNCH & DINNER RECIPES

ENJOY ON/AFTER DAY 3...

BEEF:

Beanless Chili
Beef & Zucchini Skillet
Beefy Rice Dinner*
Brussels Sprout Stuffed
  Meatballs
Clean Pumpkin Chili
South of the Border Meatloaf
Spanish Style Cabbage
Spicy Beef Tips

CHICKEN:

Chicken Fajitas
Chicken Fiesta Salad
Garlic Lime Chicken
Slow Cooker Shredded
  Chicken
Southwest Chopped Salad
Stuffed Chicken Breast

FISH:

Baked Garlic Lemon Tilapia
Keep-It-Tight Tilapia
Lemon Dill Baked Salmon
Sassy Shrimp Cocktail
Tuna Lettuce Wraps

SOUP:

Butternut Squash Soup
Savory Onion Soup
Zucchini Soup

TURKEY:

Slow Cooker 3 Bean
  Turkey Chili
Turkey Burgers*
White Chili

VEGETARIAN:

Green Chili Veggie Burgers
Oven-Roasted Tomatoes
Slow Cooker Butternut Black
Bean Quinoa

*Enjoy on/after Day 11

BEANLESS CHILI | 2 - 4 SERVINGS

Ingredients

- 1 lb. of extra lean ground beef
- 1 onion, chopped
- 1 bell pepper, chopped
- 1 (8 oz.) can of stewed tomatoes
- 1 (8 oz.) can of tomato sauce
- 1 pkg. of low-sodium or sodium-free chili seasoning mix

Directions

1. Season and brown lean ground beef.

2. Strain well to remove extra fat.

3. Mix onion, and bell pepper, add stewed tomatoes, tomato sauce, and chili mix.

4. Simmer on low-medium heat for approximately 10 minutes.

Suddenly Slim **Recipe Box**

BEEF & ZUCCHINI SKILLET | 2 - 4 SERVINGS

Ingredients
- 1 lb. of extra lean ground beef
- 2 onions
- 3-4 medium zucchinis
- 1/4 cup of butter
- 1-2 tsp. minced garlic or garlic powder
- 1 tsp. of sea salt, pepper, onion powder, basil
- oregano and thyme, to taste
- crushed red pepper flakes, optional

Directions
1. Heat skillet over medium high heat.

2. Thinly slice onions and add to skillet.

3. Using a peeler or food processor that can julienne, slice the zucchini into "noodles" and add to skillet.

4. Cook until starting to soften.

5. Remove from the skillet and place in a baking dish.

6. Put under the broiler and cook about 7-10 minutes until desired crispness.

7. While cooking, brown the ground beef and add spices of choice.

8. Add onions/zucchini back to the skillet, mix and serve.

9. Top with any desired toppings and enjoy!

Adapted from **wellnessmama.com**

BEEFY RICE DINNER | ENJOY ON/AFTER DAY 11+
2 SERVINGS

Ingredients
- 1 lb. of lean ground beef
- 1 green bell pepper
- 1 red bell pepper
- 1 onion
- 1 tsp. extra-virgin olive oil
- 1 cup 10-minute brown rice
- McCormick's no/low-sodium Savory Seasoning, to taste
- garlic powder, to taste
- fresh diced tomatoes
- sea salt, to taste

Directions
1. Brown ground beef and drain.

2. Add veggies and sauté with seasoning and 1 tsp. of olive oil.

3. Add tomatoes, cook for about 5 minutes. While this is all cooking, cook 10-minute brown rice.

4. Add olive oil, sprinkle of sea salt, garlic powder, and McCormick's savory seasoning to the rice while cooking it.

5. Combine beef and rice mixture and serve.

Suddenly Slim **Recipe Box**

118

BRUSSELS SPROUT STUFFED MEATBALLS
2 - 4 SERVINGS

Ingredients
- 2 lbs. extra lean ground beef
- 12 Brussels sprouts
- 1 white/yellow onion, chopped and browned
- 2 cups chopped spinach
- 1 tbsp. butter, optional
- sea salt, pepper, and Italian seasoning, to taste

Directions
1. Preheat oven to 375°F.
2. Mix together seasonings, meat, onions, and spinach, to form patties.
3. If desired, add butter to each sprout and place sprout in the middle of each patty. Work it into a ball around sprout.
4. Place in baking dish and bake at 375°F for 40 minutes.

Submitted by **Ashley Rudolph**

CLEAN PUMPKIN CHILI | 3 - 4 SERVINGS

Ingredients
- 1 lb. lean ground beef, browned
- 1 (15.5 oz.) can of chili beans, undrained
- 1 (15.5 oz.) can black beans, drained
- 1 (32 oz.) can of tomatoes, undrained
- 1 (15 oz.) can of pumpkin, no sugar added

Directions
1. Place all ingredients in slow cooker on low for 8-10 hours or high for 3-4 hours.

Submitted by **Coletta Hakenewerth**

SOUTH OF THE BORDER MEATLOAF | 4 SERVINGS

Ingredients
- 1 1/2 lbs. lean ground beef
- 1 tsp. fresh ground pepper
- 1 (10oz.) can Ro*Tel tomatoes and green chilies
- 1/4 cup celery, chopped
- 1/4 cup bell pepper, chopped
- 1/3 cup fresh mushrooms, chopped
- 1/4 cup onion, chopped
- 1 tbsp. fresh parsley, chopped
- 1/2 tsp. oregano
- 1 clove garlic, minced
- 1/2 cup no/low-sodium beef broth
- 1/2 cup salsa
- 1 tbsp. salt
- 1 tsp. pepper

Directions
1. Preheat oven to 350°F.

2. Mix all ingredients, except salsa, together.

3. Divide into four equal amounts and form each into a loaf shape.

4. Bake at 350°F. until done, about 20-30 minutes.
   Do not overcook or meat will dry out.

5. Heat salsa over low heat or microwave until warm.
   Pour over meatloaf before serving.

* If you have a pan with a roasting rack, line bottom of pan with
  foil and spray rack with cooking spray for easier clean up.

Submitted by **Coletta Hakenewerth**

SPANISH STYLE CABBAGE | 2 - 4 SERVINGS

Ingredients
- 1 lb. lean ground beef, venison, or turkey
- 1/2 head of cabbage chopped
- 1 medium onion sliced length wise
- 1 packet no/low-sodium taco seasoning
- 2 tbsp. butter
- 1 can Ro*Tel

Directions
1. Brown meat, drain.
2. Sauté chopped cabbage and onion in butter until tender.
3. Add the meat to the cabbage and onion, sprinkle taco seasoning all over.
4. Add can of Ro*Tel and half a can of water.
5. Stir well and simmer until liquid is absorbed.

Submitted by **Melissa Johnson**

SPICY BEEF TIPS | 1 SERVING

Ingredients
- 1 cup no/low-sodium, fat-free beef broth
- 1/2 lb. lean steak, cut 1/4" thick
- 1 tbsp. real butter, no-salt-added
- 1 tbsp. onion, minced
- 1/8 tsp. cayenne pepper
- 1 clove garlic, minced
- 1/2 tsp. sea salt
- 1/4 tsp. cinnamon
- 1 tsp. dry mustard
- 1/4 tsp. celery seed
- 1/4 tsp. chili powder

Directions
1. Brown strips in hot butter in large skillet add mixture of remaining ingredients, stir to mix.
2. Cover and simmer for 25-30 min or until meat is tender.

Days 11+ Option:
Serve over 1 cup baked brown rice. See recipe under sides.

Submitted by **Reneé Eads**

CHICKEN FAJITAS | 1 SERVING

Ingredients
- 1 (6-8 oz.) chicken breast, cut into thin strips
- 1 onion, sliced and separated into strips
- 1 green & red bell pepper, sliced
- 6-8 sliced mushrooms, optional
- 1 tbsp. extra-virgin olive oil
- 1 tbsp. minced garlic
- 1 tbsp. garlic powder
- 1 tbsp. Mrs. Dash Fiesta Lime Seasoning
- 1 tbsp. lime juice, chili powder & cumin, optional or to taste
- sea salt and pepper, to taste

Directions
1. Season meat with sea salt, pepper, garlic powder, and Mrs. Dash Fiesta Lime Seasoning and cook in 1 tbsp. olive oil in skillet until almost completely done.

2. Remove from heat & cover to keep warm.

3. Add veggies & garlic to skillet. Cook until almost to desired tenderness, then add the meat back into the skillet.

4. Season all with desired amounts of seasonings and cook until meat is done and veggies are tender or caramelized to your liking.

5. You can also add in tomatoes to the veggies at the end of the cooking process if desired!

Days 11+ Option: Add 1 cup baked brown rice to the mixture after it has been blended. See recipe under sides.

Suddenly Slim **Recipe Box**

CHICKEN FIESTA SALAD | 2 SERVINGS

Ingredients
- 2 (6-8 oz.) skinless, boneless chicken breast halves, cut in 1/2 inch strips
- 1 (1.27 oz.) packet no/low-sodium dry fajita seasoning, divided
- 1 tbsp. extra-virgin olive oil
- 1 (15 oz.) can black beans, rinsed and drained
- 1/2 cup salsa
- 1 (10 oz.) package mixed salad greens
- 1 onion, chopped
- 1 tomato, cut into wedges

Directions
1. Place chicken strips in Ziploc bag.

2. Sprinkle chicken evenly with 1/2 of the fajita seasoning. Refrigerate 30 minutes.

3. Heat the olive oil in a skillet over medium heat, and cook the chicken until juices run clear; set aside.

4. In a large saucepan, mix beans, salsa, and other 1/2 of the fajita seasoning. Heat over medium heat until warm.

5. Prepare the salad by tossing the greens, onion, and tomato. Top salad with chicken and dress with the bean mixture.

Submitted by **Reneé Eads**

GARLIC LIME CHICKEN | 4 SERVINGS

Ingredients
- 4 (6-8 oz.) boneless, skinless chicken breast halves
- 3/4 tsp. sea salt
- 1/4 tsp. black pepper
- 1/4 tsp. cayenne pepper
- 1/8 tsp. paprika
- 1/4 tsp. garlic powder
- 1/8 tsp. onion powder
- 1/4 tsp. dried thyme
- 1/4 tsp. dried parsley
- 2 tbsp. butter
- 1 tbsp. extra-virgin olive oil
- 3 tbsp. lime juice

Directions
1. In a small bowl, mix together sea salt, black pepper, cayenne, paprika, garlic powder, onion powder, thyme, and parsley.

2. Sprinkle spice mixture generously on both sides of chicken breasts.

3. Heat butter and olive oil in a large skillet over medium heat.

4. Sauté chicken until golden brown, about 6 minutes on each side.

5. Sprinkle with lime juice.

6. Cook 5 minutes, stirring frequently to coat evenly with sauce.

Suddenly Slim **Recipe Box**

SLOW COOKER SHREDDED CHICKEN | 10 SERVINGS

Ingredients
- 10 (4-6 oz.) boneless, skinless chicken breast
- 1/4 cup extra-virgin olive oil
- 2 tbsp. garlic, minced
- 1 tsp. sea salt
- 1 tsp. fresh ground black pepper
- 1/2 cup no/low-sodium chicken broth

Directions
1. Place chicken in slow cooker.

2. Drizzle with olive oil being sure to coat all sides.

3. Add all seasonings.

4. Pour broth around chicken.

5. Cover and cook on low for 6-8 hours or on high for 3-4 hours.

6. Remove chicken and shred with a fork.

Adapted from **Skinny Ms.**

SOUTHWEST CHOPPED SALAD | 2 - 4 SERVINGS

Salad Ingredients
- 1 large head of romaine
- 1 can of black beans, rinsed and drained
- 1 large orange bell pepper
- 1 pint cherry tomatoes
- 1 chopped cauliflower
- 5 green onions
- 1/4 avocado

Salad Dressing Ingredients
- 1 cup loosely packed cilantro, stems removed and roughly chopped
- 1/2 avocado
- 1 tbsp. fresh lime juice (1/2 lime), more to taste
- 1-2 garlic cloves
- 1/4 cup extra-virgin olive oil
- 1 1/2 tsp. water
- 1/8 tsp. sea salt

Directions
1. For **Salad**: Finely chop romaine, bell pepper, tomatoes, and green onions. Place all ingredients in a large bowl and stir to combine. Toss with dressing.

2. For **Dressing**: Puree all ingredients in a food processor/blender until smooth. Taste and adjust seasonings, if necessary.

Submitted by **Wendy Miller**

STUFFED CHICKEN BREAST | 4 SERVINGS

Ingredients
- 4 (6-8 oz.) boneless, skinless chicken breasts
- 2 cups fresh spinach, chopped
- 1 cup fresh mushrooms, sliced
- 1/2 cup onions, chopped

Directions
1. Preheat oven to 350°F.

2. Slice pocket open in side of each chicken breast.

3. Stuff opening with spinach, mushrooms, and onions.

4. Cover baking dish and bake at 350°F for 25 minutes or until chicken is cooked throughout.

Suddenly Slim **Recipe Box**

BAKED GARLIC LEMON TILAPIA | 6 SERVINGS

Ingredients
- 6 (6-oz.) tilapia filets
- 4 cloves garlic, crushed
- 2 tbsp. butter
- 2 tbsp. fresh lemon juice
- 4 tsp. fresh parsley
- sea salt and pepper, to taste
- cooking spray

Directions
1. Preheat oven to 400°F.

2. Melt butter on a low flame in a small saucepan.

3. Add garlic and sauté on low for about 1 minute.

4. Add the lemon juice and turn off flame.

5. Spray the bottom of a baking dish lightly with cooking spray.

6. Place the fish on top and season with sea salt and pepper.

7. Pour the lemon butter mixture on the fish & top with fresh parsley.

8. Bake at 400°F until cooked, about 15 minutes.

Suddenly Slim **Recipe Box**

KEEP-IT-TIGHT TILAPIA | 4 SERVINGS

Ingredients
- 4 tilapia filets, thawed
- 1/4 cup extra-virgin olive oil
- 3 cloves garlic, minced or pressed
- 1 tsp. fresh ground black pepper
- 1 pinch cayenne pepper

- 1 tsp. paprika
- 1 tsp. ginger
- 1 tsp. oregano
- 1 tsp. dried mustard

Directions
1. Preheat oven to 400°F.
2. Line your baking sheet with parchment paper.
3. In a medium-sized bowl combine olive oil, garlic, and seasonings.
4. Dip each filet into the seasoning & place it on the baking sheet.
5. Pour any remaining seasoning over the filets and place the baking sheet in the oven.
6. Bake for 10 minutes.

Suddenly Slim **Recipe Box**

LEMON DILL BAKED SALMON | 1 SERVING

Ingredients
- 1 salmon filet
- 2 tbsp. extra-virgin olive oil
- 1 tsp. Mrs. Dash lemon pepper seasoning

- 1 tsp. garlic powder
- 1 tsp. dill weed
- sea salt, to taste

Directions
1. Preheat oven to 375°F.
2. Pour 2 tbsp. olive oil into baking dish. Dip each side of fish into olive oil then sprinkle with all seasonings.
3. Bake at 375°F, 8-10 minutes, or until flaky.

Suddenly Slim **Recipe Box**

SASSY SHRIMP COCKTAIL | 2 SERVINGS

Ingredients
- 6 large fresh or fully thawed shrimp
- 4 tbsp. salsa
- 1 tsp. horseradish
- 1 tsp. pickling spice
- 2 leaves of romaine lettuce
- 2 lemon wedges

Directions
1. Mix 4 tbsp. of salsa with 1 tsp. of horseradish and chill.

2. In a small saucepan over high heat, bring two cups of water and one rounded tbsp. of pickling spice to a rolling boil.

3. Add the shrimp and return to a boil for one and a half minutes only. Take care not to overcook.

4. Immediately cool the shrimp in cold running water and chill.

5. To serve, place 3 shrimp on each plate with romaine lettuce. Add the salsa/horseradish sauce and lemon wedge to garnish.

Submitted by **Dave Hamer**

TUNA LETTUCE WRAPS | 1 SERVING

Ingredients
- 1 (6.5 oz. can) water packed, low-sodium, albacore tuna
- 1 onion, chopped
- 1 handful of spinach
- 1 stalk of celery, chopped
- 1/4 tsp. garlic powder
- 1 tbsp. Mrs. Dash, table blend
- 2 tbsp. light Italian or light sesame ginger dressing
- 1/4 head of bib lettuce
- fresh cracked pepper and sea salt, to taste

Directions
1. Blend all ingredients together except lettuce. Scoop into bib lettuce and serve.

Days 11+ Option:
Add 1 cup baked brown rice to the mixture after it has been blended. See recipe under sides.

Submitted by **Reneé Eads**

BUTTERNUT SQUASH SOUP | 5-6 SERVINGS

Ingredients
- 1 medium to large butternut squash
- 1/2 onion, diced
- 1 tsp. garlic, minced
- 4-6 cups no/low-sodium chicken stock (enough to cover squash)
- 2 tbsp. extra-virgin olive oil
- fresh ground black pepper and sea salt, to taste

Directions
1 Sauté diced onion and garlic with 2 tbsp. olive oil.

2. Add black pepper and salt to taste.

3. Peel squash and cut up into 1" cubes.

4. Add squash to pan and sauté for 5-10 min.

5. Pour chicken stock over the squash until covered.

6. Simmer until squash is soft.

7. Remove from heat and allow to cool slightly.

8. Add to blender and purée.

Submitted by **Angela Carr**

SAVORY ONION SOUP | 5 -6 SERVINGS

Ingredients
- 1 (6 oz.) fat-free, no/low-sodium beef broth
- 1 (16 oz.) fat-free, no/low-sodium chicken broth
- 2 cups sliced onions
- 2 tsp. minced garlic
- 1 bay leaf
- fresh ground black pepper, to taste

Directions
1. In a non-stick pan, over medium-high heat, stir fry onion and garlic until the onions are tender and caramelized. A few drops of water may be added to prevent the onions from scorching.
2. When the onions are tender, add remaining ingredients.
3. Bring to a boil, then reduce heat and simmer for 10 minutes.
4. Serve 8 oz. in a warm bowl.

Submitted by **Dave Hamer**

ZUCCHINI SOUP | 1 - 2 SERVINGS

Ingredients
- 1 1/2 lbs. zucchini, halved lengthwise & sliced 1/4 inch thick
- 2 tbsp. extra-virgin olive oil
- 1 small onion, finely chopped
- sea salt and ground pepper, to taste
- 1 tbsp. unsalted butter
- 1 garlic clove, thinly sliced

Directions
1. In a large saucepan, melt the butter in the olive oil. Add the onion and garlic, season with sea salt and pepper and cook over moderately low heat, stirring frequently until softened, 7 to 8 minutes. Add the zucchini and cook, stirring frequently, until softened about 10 minutes.
2. Working in 2 batches, puree soup in blender until smooth. Return soup to saucepan and season with sea salt and pepper. Serve hot or chilled and garnish with julienned zucchini.

Submitted by **Coletta Hakenewerth**

SLOW COOKER 3 BEAN TURKEY CHILI
4 -6 SERVINGS

Ingredients
- 1.3 lb (20 oz.) fat-free ground turkey breast
- 1 small onion, chopped
- 1 (28 oz.) can no-salt-added diced tomatoes
- 1 (16 oz.) can no-salt-added tomato sauce
- 1 (4.5 oz.) can chopped chilies, drained
- 1 (15 oz.) can chickpeas, rinsed & drained
- 1 (15.5 oz.) can black beans, rinsed & drained
- 1 (15.5 oz.) can small red beans, rinsed & drained
- 2 tbsp. chili powder
- 1/2 cup water

Garnish
- 1/2 cup red onion, chopped
- 1/2 cup fresh cilantro, chopped

Directions
1. Brown turkey and onion in a medium skillet over medium high heat until cooked through.

2. Drain any fat remaining and transfer to slow cooker.

3. Add the beans, chilies, chickpeas, tomatoes, tomato sauce, and chili powder, mixing well.

4. Cook on high 6-8 hours.

5. Garnish with onions and cilantro.

Adapted Gina's Recipes from **Skinnytaste.com**

TURKEY BURGERS | 2 -4 SERVINGS

Ingredients
- 1 pkg. lean ground turkey
- 1 pkg. fresh or frozen spinach, sautéed and drained
- 1 can small box of mushrooms, sautéed and drained
- pinch nutmeg
- sea salt and pepper, to taste
- thermic burger toppings: lettuce, tomato, onion, etc.

Directions
1. Combine ingredients in large bowl.

2. Form into burgers.

3. Sauté a small amount of garlic with olive oil just enough to coat the pan.

4. Cook for 3 minutes on each side.

Days 11+ Option:
Serve on 1 slice of Ezekiel, pumpernickel, or whole grain rye bread with lettuce and tomato.

Suddenly Slim **Recipe Box**

WHITE CHILI | 2 - 4 SERVINGS

Ingredients
- 1 lb. ground turkey
- 1 tsp. cumin
- 1 small can chopped green chilis
- 1 small yellow bell pepper
- 1 cup no/low-sodium, chicken broth
- 1 jalapeno (optional, for spice)
- 2 tbsp. chili powder
- 1 tsp. black pepper
- 1 tsp. garlic powder
- 1 onion, chopped
- 1 tbsp. minced garlic

Directions
1. Cook turkey, chili powder, cumin, black pepper, garlic powder, onion, and minced garlic in deep skillet until meat is done.
2. Add bell pepper and cook until desired tenderness.
3. Add broth and simmer for 30 minutes.

Days 11+ Option:
Add 1 cup of pinto beans or great northern beans. This will double your protein content, so adjust the serving size accordingly.

Submitted by **Reneé Eads**

GREEN CHILI VEGGIE BURGERS | 2 - 4 SERVINGS

Ingredients
- 2 onions, minced
- 3 cloves of garlic, minced
- 1 (15 oz.) can chickpeas, rinsed and thoroughly drained
- 1-2 tbsp. extra-virgin olive oil
- 1 (4oz.) can mild green chilies
- 1 tsp. cumin
- 1 tsp. chili powder
- 1 lime, juiced
- 1 handful cilantro, chopped
- 1/2-cup breadcrumbs
- sea salt and pepper to taste

Directions
1. Preheat oven to 375°F.

2. Heat large skillet on medium heat, once hot add 1 tbsp. olive oil, onion and garlic, sauté, stirring frequently until soft and translucent, about 1-2 mins.

3. When done add mixture to mixing bowl, then add chickpeas and use fork to mash/mix up. A little texture is ok, but you want only a few whole chickpeas remaining.

4. Add remaining ingredients, including 1-2 tbsp. oil, and stir/mash together. You want to form moldable dough.

5. Divide evenly into burgers (I used a 1/2 cup to make slider size patties)

6. Heat that same skillet up again; once hot, add a thin layer of olive oil to your skillet, and cook 3-4 mins on each side.

7. For a firmer burger put them in the oven at 375°F for 15-20 minutes.

Submitted by **Danette Jones**

OVEN-ROASTED TOMATOES | 8 SERVINGS

Ingredients
- 2 1/2 lbs. red and/or yellow cherry, grape, and/or other miniature tomatoes, such as roma
- 2 tbsp. extra-virgin olive oil
- 2 tbsp. balsamic vinegar
- 2 cloves garlic, minced
- 1/2–1 tsp. sea salt
- 1/2 tsp. freshly ground black pepper
- 2 tbsp. snipped fresh basil
- whole wheat bread slices

Directions
1. Preheat oven to 400°F.

2. Line a 13×9×2-inch baking pan with foil. Remove and discard stems from tomatoes; wash tomatoes. Pat tomatoes dry with paper towels. Arrange tomatoes in a single layer in prepared pan. In a small bowl whisk together olive oil, vinegar, garlic, sea salt, and pepper. Pour over tomatoes and toss tomatoes to coat.

3. Bake, uncovered, in a 400°F oven 14 to 18 minutes or just until the tomatoes are soft and skins begin to split, gently stirring once.

4. Transfer the tomatoes to a shallow serving bowl. Drizzle the balsamic mixture from the pan over the tomatoes. Sprinkle with snipped basil. Serve warm or at room temperature.

Days 11+ Option:
If you like, garnish with fresh basil sprigs and serve with bread to dip in the vinegar mixture.

Suddenly Slim **Recipe Box**

SLOW COOKER BUTTERNUT SQUASH
AND **BLACK BEAN QUINOA** | 2 SERVINGS

Ingredients
- 3 cups butternut squash, diced
- 1 cup red onion, diced
- 1 cup bell peppers, diced
- 3 garlic cloves, minced
- 1 (15 oz.) can organic black beans
- 1 (28 oz.) can of fire roasted tomatoes
- 3–4 cups no/low-sodium vegetable broth
- 2 tbsp. tomato paste
- 1/2 cup uncooked quinoa
- 1 tbsp. chili powder
- 2 tsp. cumin
- 2 tsp. paprika
- 1 tsp. coriander
- 1/2 tsp. cayenne, more or less to taste
- sea salt & pepper to taste

Directions
1. Add all ingredients into a slow cooker (starting with just 3 cups of broth). Turn on high and cook for 4 hours, turn down to low and continue to cook until ready to serve. If too thick, stir in another 1/2–1 cup of water.

Adapted from **simplyquinoa.com**

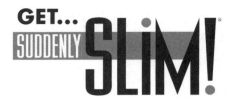

BREADS & GRAINS RECIPES

ENJOY ON/AFTER DAY 11...

Baked Brown Rice
Perfect Brown Rice
Quinoa Tabbouleh
Slow Cooker Minestrone with Quinoa

BAKED BROWN RICE | 2 SERVINGS

Ingredients
- 1 1/2 cups brown rice, medium or short grain
- 1 tbsp. unsalted butter
- 2 1/2 cups water
- 1 tsp. sea salt

Directions
1. Preheat the oven to 375 degrees F.
2. Place the rice into an 8-inch square glass baking dish.
3. Bring the water, butter, and salt just to a boil in a covered saucepan.
4. Once the water boils, pour it over the rice, stir to combine, and cover the dish tightly with heavy-duty aluminum foil.
5. Bake on the middle rack of the oven for 1 hour.
6. After 1 hour, remove cover and fluff the rice with a fork.

Adapted from **Alton Brown**

PERFECT BROWN RICE | 1 SERVING

Ingredients
- 1 cup brown rice, medium or long-grain
- 12 cups water
- sea salt, to taste

Directions
1. Rinse rice in strainer under cold water for 30 seconds. Bring 12 cups water to boil in large pot with tight fitting lid over high heat.
2. Add rice, stir it once, and boil uncovered for 30 minutes
3. Pour rice into strainer over the sink.
4. Let rice drain for 10 seconds, then return it to the pot, off the heat.
5. Cover the pot and set aside to allow the rice to steam for 6. minutes. Uncover the rice, fluff with fork and season with sea salt.

Brown rice tastes best when it has been boiled and drained like pasta, and then steamed in the small amount of moisture that remains in the pot. The boiling cooks the rice, while the subsequent steaming allows the grains to retain their integrity and come out light and fluffy.

Adapted from **Saveur.com**

Perfect Rice Variations:
(add different seasonings to create a new meal)

Mexican: cilantro and lime

Latin: pureed garlic, onion, cilantro, tomatoes and cumin

Peruvian: chopped cilantro, cumin, onions

Chinese: light, sodium reduced soy, sesame oil, ginger, & scallions

Fried Rice: 1 egg scrambled, green onion,

Spicy: red pepper flakes, chili powder, and diced jalapenos

Indian: bay leaves, cinnamon, cumin, cardamom, peppercorns, cloves and butter

QUINOA TABBOULEH | 2 SERVINGS

Ingredients
- 1 3/4 cup water
- 1/2 cup roma tomato
- 1/4 cup fresh lemon juice
- 2 tbsp. extra-virgin olive oil
- 1/4 tsp. fresh ground pepper
- 1 cup uncooked quinoa
- 1/2 cup chopped parsley
- 2 tbsp. chopped green onion
- 1/2 tsp. sea salt

Directions
1. Combine water and uncooked quinoa in a medium saucepan. Bring to boil.
2. Cover and reduce heat, simmering for 20 minutes or until all liquid is absorbed.
3. Remove from heat and fluff with a fork.
4. Stir in remaining ingredients.
5. Cover and let stand for 1 hour.
6. Serve chilled or at room temperature.

Adapted from **Cooking Light**

SLOW COOKER MINESTRONE WITH QUINOA
4 - 6 SERVINGS

Ingredients
- 1 cup yellow onion, minced
- 1 cup celery, chopped
- 1 1/2 cup zucchini, diced
- 2 cloves garlic, minced
- 1 (28 oz.) can of no/low-sodium diced tomatoes
- 2 cups frozen green beans
- 1 tsp. dried basil
- 1/2 tsp. dried oregano
- 1/2 tsp. dried rosemary
- 1/2 tsp. dried thyme
- 1/2 tsp. sea salt
- 1 (14 oz.) can cannellini beans, drained and rinsed
- 1 (14 oz.) can red kidney beans, drained and rinsed
- 6 cups no/low-sodium vegetable broth
- 3/4 cup dry quinoa
- fresh parsley, chopped, for topping

Directions
1. Place everything in slow cooker, except for parsley.
2. Cook on low for 6 to 8 hours.
3. Serve with fresh parsley.

Adapted from **RachelCooks.com**

CONCLUSION

In closing, while you have done this for yourself, I cannot thank you enough for buying my book. My life's work has been devoted to helping others, such as yourself. It never ceases to amaze me what people can do when they put their mind to a goal. In this, our common goal to Get *Suddenly Slim*, we are aligned. If you like what you've read, join the movement, and share Get *Suddenly Slim* with those you love most. There can be no greater gift than that of health.

Do you have a success story? I want to hear it. Share your weight loss and wellness successes with me! Have a pair of jeans that used to be "snug," but now they are too big? I want to see it! I am active on our social media accounts, see below, and would love for you to submit your success stories to **Lee@ GetSuddenlySlim.com**. I will happily share your successes with our community, especially if it helps just one more person take their first step toward improving their life, so they can finally Get *Suddenly Slim*.

facebook.com/**GetSuddenlySlimBook/timeline**

@GetSuddenlySlim

Lee@GetSuddenlySlim.com

Phyllisor Sam.firstfitness.com

Phyllis & Sam Orr
231-597-0170

144